Health, Technology and Society

Series Editors: **Andrew Webster**, University of York, UK and **Sally Wyatt**, Royal Netherlands Academy of Arts and Sciences, The Netherlands

Titles include:

Ellen Balka, Eileen Green and Flis Henwood (*editors*)
GENDER, HEALTH AND INFORMATION TECHNOLOGY IN CONTEXT

Courtney Davis and John Abraham (*editors*)
UNHEALTHY PHARMACEUTICAL REGULATION
Innovation, Politics and Promissory Science

Gerard de Vries and Klasien Horstman (*editors*)
GENETICS FROM LABORATORY TO SOCIETY
Societal Learning as an Alternative to Regulation

Alex Faulkner
MEDICAL TECHNOLOGY INTO HEALTHCARE AND SOCIETY
A Sociology of Devices, Innovation and Governance

Herbert Gottweis, Brian Salter and Catherine Waldby
THE GLOBAL POLITICS OF HUMAN EMBRYONIC STEM CELL SCIENCE
Regenerative Medicine in Transition

Roma Harris, Nadine Wathen and Sally Wyatt (*editors*)
CONFIGURING HEALTH CONSUMERS
Health Work and the Imperative of Personal Responsibility

Jessica Mesman
MEDICAL INNOVATION AND UNCERTAINTY IN NEONATOLOGY

Mike Michael and Marsha Rosengarten
INNOVATION AND BIOMEDICINE
Ethics, Evidence and Expectation in HIV

Nelly Oudshoorn
TELECARE TECHNOLOGIES AND THE TRANSFORMATION OF HEALTHCARE

Nadine Wathen, Sally Wyatt and Roma Harris (*editors*)
MEDIATING HEALTH INFORMATION
The Go-Betweens in a Changing Socio-Technical Landscape

Andrew Webster (*editor*)
NEW TECHNOLOGIES IN HEALTH CARE
Challenge, Change and Innovation

Andrew Webster (*editor*)
THE GLOBAL DYNAMICS OF REGENERATIVE MEDICINE
A Social Science Critique

Health, Technology and Society
Series Standing Order ISBN 978-1-4039-9131-7 hardback
(*outside North America only*)

You can receive future titles in this series as they are published by placing a standing order. Please contact your bookseller or, in case of difficulty, write to us at the address below with your name and address, the title of the series and the ISBN quoted above.

Customer Services Department, Macmillan Distribution Ltd, Houndmills, Basingstoke, Hampshire RG21 6XS, England

---

Innovation and Biomedicine

Ethics, Evidence and Expectation in HIV

Mike Michael
University of Sydney, Australia

and

Marsha Rosengarten
Goldsmiths, University of London, UK

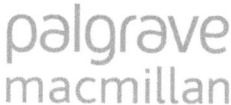

First published 2013 by
PALGRAVE MACMILLAN

Palgrave Macmillan in the UK is an imprint of Macmillan Publishers Limited, registered in England, company number 785998, of Houndmills, Basingstoke, Hampshire RG21 6XS.

Palgrave Macmillan in the US is a division of St Martin's Press LLC, 175 Fifth Avenue, New York, NY 10010.

Palgrave Macmillan is the global academic imprint of the above companies and has companies and representatives throughout the world.

Palgrave® and Macmillan® are registered trademarks in the United States, the United Kingdom, Europe and other countries

ISBN: 978–0–230–30267–9

This book is printed on paper suitable for recycling and made from fully managed and sustained forest sources. Logging, pulping and manufacturing processes are expected to conform to the environmental regulations of the country of origin.

A catalogue record for this book is available from the British Library.

A catalog record for this book is available from the Library of Congress.

Contents

Acknowledgements

This book is the fruit of a five-year collaboration, more or less. Along the way, we have published several papers and chapters and, while this present volume differs substantially from all of these, there are inevitable echoes. The most relevant previous pieces are Michael, M. and Rosengarten, M. (2012a) 'HIV, Globalization and Topology: Of Prepositions and Propositions', *Theory, Culture & Society*; Rosengarten, M. and Michael, M. (2009a) 'Rethinking the Bioethical Enactment of Drugged Bodies: On the Paradoxes of Using Anti-HIV Drug Therapy as a Technology for Prevention', *Science as Culture*; Rosengarten, M. and Michael, M. (2009b) 'The Performative Function of Expectations in Translating Treatment to Prevention: The Case of HIV Pre-exposure Prophylaxis or PrEP', *Social Science & Medicine*; and Michael, M. and Rosengarten, M. (forthcoming) *Quantitative Objects and Qualitative Things: Ethics and HIV Biomedical Prevention* in *Objects and Materials. A Routledge Companion*.

The collaboration, itself, has been made possible through the contributions of many others. We would like especially to thank the various participants who have agreed to speak to us, or else have provided us with various empirical materials. In particular, we wish to thank our anonymous informants along with many members of the HIV field and notably Keith Alcorn, Judy Auerbach, Carlos Cáceres, Gus Cairns, Julie Davids, Robert Grant, Ade Fakoya, Kimberly Gray, Karyn Kaplan, Mark Harrington, Martin Holt, Susan Kippax, Albert Liu, Dean Murphy, Eric Mykhalovskiy, Susie McLean, Cheryl Overs, Kate MacQueen, Kane Race, Fiona Samuels, Niamh Stephenson and Mitchell Warren. We would like to acknowledge the support of the Sociology Department at Goldsmiths, University of London and latterly the Department of Sociology and Social Policy at the University of Sydney. Inevitably, we will fail to thank all the many colleagues who have contributed in one way or another to the development of this book – a partial list includes Vikki Bell, Mariam Fraser, Bill Gaver, Mick Halewood, Tobie Kerridge, Celia Lury, Noortje Marres, David Oswell, Nirmal Puwar and Alex Wilkie.

Mike Michael would like to thank Bethan, Nye and Yanna Rees for their unstinting forbearance, love and support.

Marsha Rosengarten would like to thank Cath Le Couteur for an immense amount of things, most of all for being there.

1
Introduction: Setting a Scene

It is a commonplace to worry about the pace of innovation in biomedicine. From the perspective of some actors, innovation moves too quickly, throwing up complex regulatory issues and ethical dilemmas that are sometimes barely tractable. For others, innovation cannot take place fast enough: in the here and now, there are lives to be saved and there is suffering to be eased. Often these two contrasting apprehensions toward biomedical innovation reside simultaneously in a single actor (whether that actor be individual or collective). This ambivalence reflects the contradictory character of much that passes for biomedical innovation. With the development and arrival of a new drug, technology, procedure or intervention, not only might lives be saved, but they can also be endangered at one and the same time.

However, portraying the concerns associated with biomedical innovation in terms of such ambivalence misses the point on several levels. Or rather, it frames the issue in a very particular way that reflects, mediates and enacts a series of ontological, epistemological, political, social and ethical perspectives. By way of initial illustration, let us focus on the possible negative impacts of a new therapy. Immediately, we might note that it is not only the health of bare lives that is potentially placed at risk. This intervention can also negatively affect, for example, local and national communities, civil rights, economic opportunity, wider health system provision or particular types of gendered relations. To make this observation is to begin to shift our understanding of that intervention. Ontologically, it is not simply constituted of its material composition and technical properties (for example, such and such a pharmaceutical compound, such and such an effect on a disease entity or such and such side-effects on a human body) but emerges out of a nexus of complex, multifarious and shifting relations that includes a range of material, individual, community, institutional, policy and political actors. Epistemologically, an intervention is not knowable simply through the assumptions that inform bioscientific and biomedical techniques (for example, the objectivity of randomized controlled trials) but through a model of knowing, or engagement, that aims to capture the situatedness, relationality, emergence and performativity of a representation of a biomedical intervention. Such interventions are not politically and socially neutral, or even complicated in the sense that there are very many political and social factors to be taken into account in order to develop, deploy and assess an intervention. Rather, these social and political elements are complex in that they relate to each other recursively: the borders between social categories or political actors come in and out of focus in sometimes unusual and unexpected ways. Ethically, the intervention is judged in relation to a set of impacts that extends far beyond the individual or the statistically aggregated body. But further, this process of ethical judgement that identifies and compares positive and negative effects has its own particular trajectory. It reflects, mediates and enacts a practice of ethics which folds into and contributes to the ontological, epistemological, social and political emergence of the intervention.

Hopefully, the foregoing should have provided a preliminary sense of a series of interconnected relations – ontological, epistemological, material, social, political and ethical – through which we can approach biomedical innovation. Or, to put this another way and introduce another term, we can address biomedical innovation with the aid of the notion of 'assemblage'. We shall have quite a lot to say about this idea along with a number of other supplementary concepts such as 'object' and 'thing', 'topology', 'enactment', and especially 'event'. However, what we can point out here is that this particular formulation, albeit all too vague at the moment, is not just derived from the theoretical literature. Crucially, it is also shaped by our engagement with specificities of biomedical innovation within the HIV field, and especially the randomized controlled trialling (from here on referred to as RCT or RCTs) of a pre-exposure prophylactic intervention, a pill taken every day that ostensibly decreases the risk of HIV infection (PrEP).

That is to say, our thinking on innovation and biomedicine is worked through a particular example of, in some ways, a rather unexciting innovation – a pill made up of existing drugs that can serve as a prophylactic against 'the' HIV virus. Needless to say, this does not have some of the key features of more 'exotic' innovations, most obviously those associated with cutting edge, 'high technology' biomedical research such as stem cell-based regenerative medicine (for example, the fraught regulatory quandaries and ethical dilemmas of using human embryo-derived materials, or the transformation of the clinical landscape implied in the promises associated with stem cell research). Nevertheless, the complexities entailed in, and the potential associated with, a seemingly 'simple' or 'mundane' intervention like PrEP are a match for those of any of the more 'dramatic' or 'spectacular' biomedical innovations. In other words, the divide between 'exotic' and 'mundane' biomedical innovation is highly porous.

Now, we would not wish to imply that PrEP is merely an example, an illustration, a medium – to be sure a highly consequential one – with which to work through an array of issues concerning biomedicine and innovation. Rather, we are also interested in PrEP in itself, not least because it may have a major impact on individuals, communities and nations in which the risks of HIV infection are particularly elevated. For instance, through our extended case study one of the things to which we aim to draw attention is how innovation maps onto global asymmetries in wealth and medical infrastructure. Ironically, as we shall detail at some length, an asymmetry such as the effects of impoverished medical provision are not only the targets of innovations such as PrEP but also, within the parameters of practices specific to the RCT testing of interventions, a pre-requisite for the realization of PrEP as an innovation. But first we must set the scene by presenting a preliminary historical backdrop to the emergence of PrEP.

HIV and PrEP: a testing backstory

In July 2012, the United States Food and Drug Administration (FDA) approved the use of daily oral PrEP consisting of two antiretroviral drugs Tenofovir (TDF) and Emtricitabine (FTC).[1] The two drugs were already approved for use in treating existing HIV infections but their officially approved use as a means of preventing infection confirmed that they could now become medically available for those of HIV negative status. That is, they could be legally prescribed for those not infected with HIV but for whom there is the possibility of sexual exposure to the virus. FDA approval followed a review of laboratory-based evidence and a series of RCTs, which we discuss throughout the book. United States approval is likely to pave the way for a number of other countries to consider the implementation of PrEP. However, the issues raised by PrEP implementation are complex and the response to these in many ways shows a field grappling with the use of costly and potentially toxic antiretroviral drugs for widespread prevention purposes. In this book, we review some of the history of PrEP, drawing on various articles and reports that reflect but also – as our analysis will consider – have participated in the emergence in PrEP. In many respects we believe that the understanding of PrEP by the HIV field – including its promise, challenges and, for some, its wrongheadedness (where it is considered as the wrong approach to prevention) – can be traced to the manner of its development.

Although the first round of PrEP RCTs in the countries of Cambodia and Cameroon failed due to controversy about their ethics (and heated debate continues over the validity of a RCT with injecting drug users (IDUs) in Thailand that was set up at the same time), such controversy did not generate what we regard as any sort of radical rethinking. Specifically, the field did not draw on these cases to interrogate seriously the research technology of the RCT, the ethics of conducting RCTs in low and middle income countries or, crucially, standard distinctions between 'behavioural' and 'biomedical' intervention. Instead, a 'coming together' was engineered by the International AIDS Society (IAS) funded by the philanthropic organization Bill & Melinda Gates Foundation (see IAS, 2005) and, separately but with many of the same participants, by UNAIDS (2006). This 'coming together' involved large scale consultations and some weighty reports that ultimately concluded with statements of commitment to greater community consultation and participation in the planning of trials. The reports, in particular, placed emphasis on the need to inform and provide follow-up care for trial participants (see Rosengarten and Michael, 2009b).

Of course, we do not wish to imply any insincerity on the part of scientific stakeholders, that is, the trialists and their sponsors, or that the community stakeholders were in any way ineffectual in putting forward their concerns, or that community consultation and participation have no place. Nevertheless, we can suggest from a reading of such documents (as well as numerous other published materials that ensued in the wake of the early controversy) that little, if any, challenge was made to the technology of the RCT and the bioethics associated with it. In the absence of an appropriately interrogative engagement with RCTs and bioethics, one upshot has been that the field generally enacts PrEP as a singular chemoprophylaxis dependent on user adherence – a framing that comes up in almost all recent literature on PrEP. This seems to miss out not only on much of the complexity of PrEP and its testing and implementation, but also on the potential traction that PrEP might have with its various users. It thus seems to us even more imperative to revisit the work of the RCT and bioethics.

To put this in slightly different terms, what we have here is a story of multiple actors (including international research funders, international regulatory agencies, scientific experts, and articulate, media-savvy protestors) whose efforts have generated an intervention but one that in many respects confounds those who must decide on its take up. We also have a story of the tragic need for more effective prevention. Yet the very question of what makes for effective prevention, is precisely what remains to be fully explored.

In 2006, a publication first-authored by Inge Derdelinckx (and including amongst its listed authors the prominent scientist Mark Wainberg and consultant for the IAS report on PrEP discussed above, Yasmin Halima), contained the statement:

> In 2004, almost 5 million people became newly infected with HIV, emphasising the continuous need for effective prevention strategies...behavioural interventions [condoms, abstinence] may not be able to curb the HIV epidemic as much as needed.... (Derdelinckx et al., 2006:1999)

Here we refer to the statement as not only indicative of a continuing epidemic but also as illustrative of how the HIV field is enacted through the entrenched distinction between 'behavioural' and 'biomedical' interventions that, in itself, has significant implications for the development of PrEP. The distinction of 'behavioural' and 'biomedical' is readily assumed to map to the disciplinary divide of social sciences and biomedical sciences. Yet it is equally plausible that the disciplinary divide has generated the distinction. Although it is clear that the authors doubt that the use of condoms or abstinence from sex are sufficiently viable strategies for preventing HIV transmission, they do not consider that all forms of intervention involve social practices (even a vaccine requires scientists doing things collectively and users actively accessing it) and that a prevention pill, especially, will involve 'behaviour', as they put it (Kippax and Stephenson, 2012). In succinct terms, a prevention pill acquires its capacity to be so only through use, which inevitably entails social relations and practices (which are also, of course, sociomaterial). Yet, as we shall see, the RCT is not designed to investigate this. Indeed, it seems designed to avoid inquiry into what makes an intervention effective by distinguishing what is 'effective' from what can be statistically demonstrated as 'efficacious'.[2]

So, with PrEP, we find RCTs are designed to establish the preventative capacity of the drugs while excluding much of what is involved in their use (and hence in the accomplishment of prevention); this follows, we have suggested, from the disciplinary distinction between the 'behavioural' or social and the 'biomedical'. Accordingly, statistical estimates of the efficacy of PrEP have been calculated, to date, by collecting surveillance data from RCT participants about their dosing, and also in some cases about their sexual activity. Important here is the comparison between what people report about dosing and what drug levels in their blood show. If drug levels are low in an individual's blood, this is used to explain lack of 'efficacy': the lack of drug impact is put down to insufficient levels of the drug in the blood. And yet, this excludes from consideration why an individual might not dose as required in the first place – our basic point is that surely users' dosing (or not dosing) is an element key to whether PrEP can become a pre-exposure prophylaxis or not.

The bifurcated nature of prevention and PrEP RCTs that can be found across much of the HIV field and which reflects and mediates a relatively uninterrogated notion of what is effective, directs us to the question of ethics. How is it possible for millions of dollars to be expended on RCTs and yet so few to be spent on research addressed to the complexities of everyday negotiation of HIV risk (see, for example, Peters et al., 2010)?

For the HIV field, bioethics in the form of a set of principles is set out in various UNAIDS and WHO reports. The principles themselves are derived from moral philosophy and are specifically enshrined in the Helsinki Declaration[3] with adjustments to address concerns raised in response to HIV RCTs in low and middle-income countries. These sorts of RCTs are commonly referred to as 'offshore RCTs' to underscore the qualitatively different health and medical contexts in such countries compared to that of the trial sponsor. Indeed the disparity between the sponsor's country and what was proposed for the early PrEP trials in Cambodia, Cameroon and Thailand can be said to have, at least in part, mobilized opposition to the trials by local groups who expressed concern that the trials were unethical. Some even queried whether the trialists would carry out such trials on their 'own' people, their own family members (WNU, 2004; Rosengarten and Michael, 2009a).

We will discuss this controversy in some detail in this chapter and again in Chapters 5 and 7 where it will be enacted in different ways. For immediate purposes, it will be useful to set out how the undertaking of 'offshore HIV trials' generates an ethical dilemma or paradox. Different accounts provide contradictory data on how a trial affects perceptions of HIV. On the one hand, some suggest that a trial may engender 'risk compensation' by creating a false sense of security about HIV risk due to the promise of a new technology. On the other, some claim that trials actually improve community awareness of the protective value of existing measures such as the use of condoms (Paxton, 2012:559). But even where trials are able to improve community awareness of HIV risk and to increase the capacity to implement health and medical measures, there remains the possibility that trials may affect health status in the long term by adding to the burden on local medical resources:

> Epidemiologically, they are the people with the greatest need for effective prevention; statistically, they also present the most efficient opportunity to test interventions but the poverty and disempowerment that generate vulnerability to HIV infection also serve as barriers to medical care and services. Thus, the people most appropriate for enrollment in international HIV prevention trials are also the people least likely to have access to HIV treatment and care in their local communities. (MacQueen et al., 2007:554)

Our point is that HIV prevention, as articulated by Derdelinckx et al. (2006) cited above, can set in train a series of interconnected approaches that actively exclude from consideration the complex way in which transmission and its prevention by specific interventions play out in different settings. What we suggest in our review of PrEP is that new ways of problematizing HIV, prevention and treatment are required and that a reworking of the existing problematic requires conceptual tools appropriate to this task. Indeed, throughout this book we set ourselves the task of contesting many of the distinctions that have become commonplace in social scientific as well as in biomedical scientific thinking. Of course, thinking is itself not a practice that can be sequestered from material practice. We try to show that the framing in terms of distinct stable entities – including PrEP but also subjects, bodies, drugs and trials – fails to address the complexity of sociomaterial efforts to achieve ethically effective interventions. Put simply, if prevention is to take place – in this instance through the uptake of PrEP – it must perform an alignment of sorts with the sociomaterial relations and dynamics that characterize those for whom it is intended. PrEP's controversial status cannot be disentangled from the technology of the 'efficacy-testing' RCT and the legitimation of this by a particular version of bioethics. In sum, the technical and social warrants that are mobilized for RCTs in their current form (where only a delimited set of effects are of concern) exclude precisely those elements that characterize the everyday use of the candidate medical intervention – elements that variously flow into, but also from, the candidate intervention's use.

Studying and theorizing PrEP

Needless to say, the historical sketch above is by no means innocent. Indeed, to write 'a history' of the HIV/AIDS crisis and the biomedical response to it is a highly problematic undertaking for, as with any history, it is in principle always a site of contention and a text open to revision. Nevertheless, it can serve as a semi-stable backdrop against which we set out our detailed discussions of PrEP, even while our recounting of PrEP serves to, more or less subtly, re-write that history.

In thinking about PrEP in this way, we situate it in relation to a range of empirical settings, most obviously different offshore RCTs, and a series of discussions about the ethics of those trials. On one level, we might say that we are following PrEP as it moves from one setting to another – say, from particular ethical discussions about its testing through specific RCTs to the ways in which such testing of PrEP was seen by particular HIV activists to raise enormous political problems. In this historical narrative of contrasts, the meaning of PrEP is being contested. More specifically the ethical and political status of PrEP is rendered contentious: it is some 'object' that can be seen as EITHER ethically sound OR as politically suspect.

However, this account makes a number of assumptions that are not always helpful. Here are three such assumptions – more will be unravelled as we move through the book.

Firstly, there is a division between facts and values. As such, an intervention such as PrEP might be deemed controversial because divergent assessments are made of it: it might be seen as both ethically robust and politically suspect. However, these assessments attach to what is otherwise regarded as the pre-existing and stable object of PrEP. The disadvantages of this familiar formulation are manifold as we shall show in detail throughout the book. Suffice it to note for the moment that the 'object' that is PrEP is infused with the ethical and political (for example, why concoct, produce and promote this rather than another sort of prophylaxis?) and the ethical and political is suffused with claims about facts (for example, the nature of at-risk bodies, or the sustainability of local health systems). This sort of fact–value distinction tends to obscure the complexity – the heterogeneity of composition – of the issues at stake in controversies over biomedical innovation.

Secondly, there is an assumption that there is such a singular, abstracted 'object' as PrEP that lies beyond its multiple instantiations (for example, the ethically robust PrEP; the politically contentious PrEP). Simplistically, we might ask how we would access such an abstracted 'object' as PrEP except through its individual manifestation. More interestingly, we might ask how PrEP is emergent and relational – how it is 'event-ualized', that is to say, made manifest in particular events in which many entities and relations are brought together (bodies, science, ethics, health workers, pills etc.) in varying configurations or 'assemblages'. In brief, PrEP is constituted in and through its relations and, in a sense, it is 'innovated' anew as these configurations of relations shift and change. One of the interesting properties of this formulation is that we can explore not only how the different PrEPs clash, but also how they articulate, how they are managed, and also how they feed off and into each other in often highly complex, indeed ironic, ways.

Thirdly, there might be some disquiet over the assumption that it is feasible simply to follow PrEP as it emerges in relation to divergent actors and agents, along the way providing disinterested accounts of its various event-uations. This would presuppose that our own analytic, ethical and political (these should all be hyphenated of course – we would not want to reproduce the fact–value divide) accounts did not bring together their own set of relations that event-uate our own particular versions of PrEP. The issue here is how we write accounts of PrEP while acknowledging that these accounts themselves entail very specific event-uations.

Methodologically, this raises an intriguing prospect. Analytically, we might be interested in charting aspects of the 'proliferation' of PrEPs and the complexities of these PrEPs' interconnections. A key ethical and political implication of this is, as hinted at above, to show how in articulating these various PrEPs – some of which will contrast greatly with one another – and in exposing them to each other, we can find new event-uations of PrEP, new formulations marked by what we shall later call 'inventive problem-making'. However, in charting this proliferation, we ourselves are event-uating PrEP in numerous ways, drawing not only on our data (for example, interviews and participant observations, numerous archival and media materials) but also on particular theoretical problematics or frameworks. For instance, the PrEP that is analysed through an interest in the promises that are made for it (here we draw upon the sociology of expectations literature) differs from the PrEP that is analysed in terms of the role of bioethics (here we draw on critical discussions of how contemporary ethics tends to impoverish the understandings of, and responses to, the issues raised by RCTs) which, in turn, is different from the PrEP that is analysed in relation to the globalizing representations of HIV (here we draw on recent applications of topology in social science).

In our view, what is methodologically interesting here, is that these three event-uations of PrEP might draw on the 'very same' selection of data (for example, a specific report on the relation of ethics to the implementation of RCTs under a particular set of local social and medical circumstances). This does not mean we have somehow played fast and loose with the data, but to acknowledge that the data are themselves event-uated: as they become embroiled in different relations (in this case, different theoretical or conceptual framings), so they 'become' otherwise. The significance and signification of a selection or body of data is, in other words, multifarious – indicative of different meanings because it emerges through different entanglements (with other data, with other issues and concerns, with other theoretical framings). As a corollary, we can also say that these different eventuations impact upon our own conceptual positions. In the writing of the book we have found that our use of terms like 'event' has had to adapt to the data with which we have engaged. In sum, we authors have become-with our objects of study. The upshot is that 'we' have consistently striven to remain attuned to the co-emergence of data and concepts: whatever conceptual coherence or theoretical rigour can be attributed to this book rests in large part on this sensibility.

Now, to return to the assumptions that inform PrEP trials: the fact–value distinction in relation to the PrEP trials and their ethical evaluation, the singularization and stabilization of the PrEP pill, the disinterested accounting of PrEP – these do not simply apply to PrEP. Over and above the intrinsic importance of PrEP as a contentious intervention in the HIV field (we do not dispute that it might save lives), PrEP serves as a challenging but fertile example through which to re-eventuate some of the complexities of the relations between biomedicine and innovation. The broader aim is, therefore, to draw on HIV and specifically PrEP as a partial means of exploring new ways of thinking biomedical innovation in general. By unpacking several of PrEP's manifold eventuations, we thus also hope to contribute to recent discussions of (how to analyse) the concurrent emergence and impact of innovative health technologies.

Structure of the book

The overarching structure of the book is rather linear. This might seem like an obvious statement but given our penchant for things emergent and topological, it is rather ironic. While, as will become apparent, there are several loops within the book as we revisit examples or draw links between different conceptual schemas, the format we have chosen is straightforward. In light of what often felt like the unwieldy complexity of the material – not least the empirical material – the least we felt we could do is to minimize the effort of reading. That was the intention – whether we have succeeded very much remains with the reader.

The next chapter provides a more detailed historical background to our case study of PrEP, situating it in relation to the broader trajectories of both HIV prevention and treatment, to the continuing development of the key biomedical tool, namely RCTs, and to the evolving role of bioethics and bioethical assessment. Thus, we present an account of how two existing drugs came to be reformulated as a potential prophylactic and the resistance this has met, and, to some extent, continues to meet. Key to this narrative account of PrEP will be the programmatic focus upon battling the HIV epidemic in low and middle income countries and how – due to epidemiological mappings of HIV incidence and prevalence – populations with high vulnerability to HIV become 'offshore' locales for the testing of new treatments or prophylactics. As we show, the place of bioethics in the enactment of such research is immensely problematic.

Our engagement with ethics is through a preliminary consideration of the controversy that surrounded the first PrEP RCTs. Although the controversy resulted in the coming together of a diverse range of actors, recourse to bioethics by all functioned to legitimate the model of the RCT *and*, by doing so, delimit the experimental possibilities of other models of field-based research. Indeed, the manner in which the early controversy has been reported contrasts to an earlier pre-antiretroviral HIV drug period of the HIV epidemic. In the latter, HIV-affected lay members of the public have been shown to be positively central to the design of effective prevention strategies (Stengers, 1997; Kippax and Race, 2003). The account we present sets up the scene for subsequently tracing how bioethics effectively endorses a particular frame – encapsulated in the RCT – that diminishes the complexity of the phenomena that comprise HIV vulnerability and, we suggest, detracts from the importance of heterogeneity for possible prevention strategies.

The initial history and analysis set out in Chapter 2 serves to raise a series of conceptual and theoretical issues that are addressed and expanded upon in Chapter 3. Here, we outline the theoretical approaches we will use to rethink the framing of PrEP, PrEP RCTs and bioethics. Thus we begin by introducing the relevant literature on innovation, especially how it is treated in relation to biomedical research. We use this as a basis from which to develop our own analytic framework.

At base, our approach regards PrEP as an object, but one that is emergent out of a nexus of relations. On this score we follow a number of contemporary scholars such as Bruno Latour, John Law and Annmarie Mol who emphasize the relationality of objects such that what they 'are' varies depending on the particular pattern of relations out of which they emerge. We situate this 'ontological multiplicity' in the context of a theory of the event which sees the various entities that contribute to the making of the object as mutually changing. Thus to study the PrEP pill is to examine, amongst other things, the mode of the RCT, the bioethics that are associated with the RCT, the virus, the RCT scientists (who will hereon also be referred to as the trialists) and the volunteers (also referred to as trial participants) – these come together and conjoin or 'concresce' in different occasions to event-uate different PrEPs. Key authors here are A.N. Whitehead, Isabelle Stengers and Mariam Fraser. In sum, taking together the various theoretical resources supplied by these scholars allows us to conduct an empirical analysis that is sensitive to the multiplicity of PrEP, to its various eventuations, and to the different patterns and distributions of relationalities that each eventuation entails.

This means that we need to think about what it is that goes into the key events of making PrEP. This, in turn, points to the need to think about other sorts of literatures relevant to such makings of PrEP. For instance, PrEP is partly constituted by the representations of the future that 'accompany' it. That is to say, PrEP is marked by the (medical) expectations that actors attempt to attach to, and derive from, a particular pill and its testing. PrEP is also constituted through the sorts of ethical arguments that are made to adhere to it, ethical arguments that are sometimes represented as having universal reach. And PrEP is enacted in relation to the circulation of materials and signs that are sometimes seen to be global, sometimes local. These are just some of the elements or prehensions (as Whitehead would say) that are entailed in sometime divergent, sometimes common event-uations of PrEP, and each implies a different literature (though these are of course themselves limited in various ways, not least by the ostensible fact that we are sociologists of sorts). So, in addressing what goes into PrEP's eventuation, we will need to address the sociology of expectations and the future, the sociology and political science of bioethics and the sociologies of globalization and spatialization. In Chapter 3 we provide introductions to these literatures.

Throughout the book, the notions of event and eventualization are key to the analysis, not least in that they allow us to explore the prospective, immanent or virtual dimensions of particular sociomaterial happenings. Drawing especially on the work of Mariam Fraser and Isabelle Stengers, we conceptualize the event as an opportunity for cautious reconsideration of the existing politics of a possible innovation such as PrEP – politics that range from more traditional forms (for example, typical modes of regulation) to more radical forms (such as protest) with various modes of engagement or participation somewhere in between. The aim here is to draw out the prospective dimensions of the eventuation of PrEP in order to open up a 'cosmopolitical space'. In this space, it becomes possible to ask how we might eventuate PrEP – and, ideally, any innovation – otherwise, in a way that allows us to practice an 'inventive problem-making' that better formulates and addresses what is at stake in such (a process of) innovation. From this grand aspiration we move to a more mundane, but no less important, report on what we actually did in order to gather our empirical material.

In Chapter 4, we examine the PrEP trials and their accompanying bioethics in order show how multiplicity and complexity of the pill are reduced in various ways. We suggest that in the course of such reduction – or what we variously call singularization and quantification – PrEP emerges as an increasingly problematic and worrying entity, not least according to those undergoing the trials. The 'offshore' trial effectively constitutes an 'experimental' population on the promise of the trial's capacity ultimately to provide what it has already determined is a biomedical benefit (Petryna, 2007). Underpinning these dynamics is a universalized approach to the complexities of health and medicine that is encapsulated in the model of the RCT. It is an approach that elevates the 'imperative' to generalize, but without giving sufficient attention to the complex local contingencies that inevitably affect HIV transmission and prevention. So, while the RCT is celebrated for its apparent ability to exclude extraneous 'social' phenomena, everyday understandings and practices involved in the actual use of this biomedical intervention will fundamentally affect its capacity for prevention.

The doability of RCTs, and their putative capacity effectively to exclude local complexity, are also partly grounded in the bioethical justification for such trials. Bioethics is, itself, narrowly framed in ways that enable very specific enactments of possibly 'unsafe' or 'harmful' biomedical effects. In other words, bioethics will be shown in the case of PrEP to 'bracket' consideration of a much wider array of matters important to users both within and beyond the trial. Put another way, we trace how PrEP, through the conjoint mechanisms of RCTs and bioethics, is 'singularized' – exorcized of its multiplicity. Moreover, we argue, that ethics is constituted as an 'external resource' to the trial: it is a means to formulating the ethics of particular RCTs along a series of pre-set criteria that cannot accommodate the individual trial's specificity. In sum, Chapter 4 focuses on the exclusionary process achieved through the inter-relations between the biomedical and bioethical techniques that come together in the design and conduct of PrEP RCTs. Conjointly, it examines the science and the ethics that enact PrEP as a 'quantitative object', eventuated as it is through a number of external, pre-existing biomedical and ethical parameters and criteria.

By contrast, Chapter 5 begins to engage with the multiplicity and complexity of PrEP which is set in contrast to the singularizing dynamics of RCT and bioethics. Although the quantitative object of PrEP appears as a self-evident entity for those developing PrEP (including policy makers and community representatives), albeit bearing immense challenges, it is also apparent that PrEP can be understood as what we call a 'qualitative' thing. In this chapter, we examine how PrEP trialists face up to, and grapple with, its ontological multiplicity – a multiplicity in which PrEP's effectiveness is anticipated to be potentially affected by a proliferation of factors and relations that encompasses genetics, body size, gender, type of exposure, black markets, medical infrastructure, private or public health funding, local gender and economic relations of power.

Further, we show how PrEP's multiplicity emerges in relation to other 'qualitative' eventuations associated with the challenges it will pose. For example, PrEP is variously implicated in the continuation of infections due to its partial-only effectiveness (AVAC, 2005:3); as a result of PrEP's status as sub-optimal form of HIV treatment if infection occurs within individuals while taking it, there is a possibility that its distribution will precipitate resistance by the virus to those HIV treatments (Hurt et al., 2011; Paxton et al., 2007: 89); PrEP's perceived status as a new prevention may lead to a possible 'risk compensation' in which condoms are used less frequently (Poynton et al., 2012:554); PrEP facilitates more autonomy for women to protect themselves against HIV alongside greater expectations that women will come to bear the responsibility for biomedical prevention (as has happened with the contraceptive pill) (Rosengarten & Michael, 2009b:1054). As if this did not complicate the eventuations of PrEPs enough, there is also considerable debate about the level of population coverage that would be required to achieve a significant reduction in infections, and the social and economic cost of this in terms of the provision of drugs but, also, of implementing regular HIV antibody testing to ensure against the possibility that people already infected do not mistakenly use PrEP (see, for example, Abbas, 2007). These multiple, inter-related, emergent expectations and suspicions are not the preserve of social scientists, or critics or activists: clearly some trialists are acutely aware of them and try to respond to them in various ways. As such we discuss the sorts of medical, political and ethical debates and arrangements that these complexities of PrEP precipitate. One of our points is that this response is hampered by commitment to a particular enactment of the RCT and its accompanying bioethics.

What this panoply of PrEPs demonstrates is that PrEP emerges in highly contingent and relational ways that are 'qualitative'. By this we mean that what PrEP 'is' cannot be adjudged against pre-existing, external criteria or parameters (regarding RCTs or bioethics, for instance) because not only many local factors (as we have noted above) intervene, but also any external standards become 'qualified' – that is, their meaning and impact are thoroughly refashioned within the particular eventuation of PrEP. In contrast to the sort of event that makes a quantitative object of PrEP in which the different factors (prehensions such as ethics, RCTs, bodies, communities, health systems etc.) are in a state of 'being together,' there is a 'becoming together' of the different factors that eventuate the qualitative thing PrEP.

Simply put, this formulation will enable us to develop further our inquiry into the relation of ethics and scientific research this time placing emphasis on complex contingency. The chapter will be based partly on the material presented in Chapter 4, but also draw on the immense range of qualitative work available on prevention that shows how different understandings and negotiations of HIV risk emerge in relation with various cultural understandings and material conditions (including food shortages, health and medical infrastructures, politics, gender relations etc.). Particularly important to our empirical analysis will be a focus on the heterogeneous phenomena found at a local level that will eventuate PrEP's effectiveness – effectiveness that is sociomaterial, encompassing both the physical prevention of HIV infection and cultural conditions under which users may engage PrEP. As we show, this has major implications for the understanding of evidence and ethics.

If Chapter 4 broadly focuses on the processes of quantification and singularization, and Chapter 5 primarily stresses the processes of qualification and multiplicity, Chapter 6 attempts to weave the two accounts together to suggest that these processes are not simply contrastive, or oppositional, or antagonistic. In doing this, we add further to the textures of PrEP by situating 'it' in relation to the globalizing and localizing dynamics that characterize (parts of) the HIV field. As such, we are interested in how PrEP and other components of the HIV field are made and remade as local or global, and how each draws upon the other: the local is enacted by drawing on the global and vice versa. In accessing these 'involuted' associations, we attempt to think topologically.

Specifically, we draw on the concept of assemblage in order to bring out some of the numerous links that tie together various eventuations of quantitative and qualitative PrEP. For instance, in protesting against the particular implementation of RCTs (that have been warranted through a quantitative, universalistic and globalizing bioethics) activists may draw in part on another quantitative, universalistic and globalizing version of ethics.

This analysis is further extended by situating PrEP in relation to other globalizing-localizing dynamics of the HIV field, especially the interactive AIDS 'clock' on the UNFPA website that 'counts' the global total number of HIV infections. While this too entails a quantification of HIV infection, it is designed as means of inspiring action against HIV, including arguably the development of PrEP. However, the interconnections amongst the clock's 'quantification' of the HIV epidemic, and the 'qualifications' of local contingencies (described in the previous chapter) are also revealed ironically to enact one another in ways that we argue may have important implications for the material politics of HIV. The chapter then examines how PrEP – topologically eventuated as medium, as product and as affect – serves in the enactment of differences and similarities across populations and practitioners, times and spaces, medical interventions and affective tactics. We end the chapter by drawing on the work of a literary theorist additionally to explore, albeit briefly, some further ironies of topological analysis.

At this point we should note that throughout Chapters 4, 5 and 6, we make extensive use of extended quotes. In part this is because we want to afford the reader the opportunity to interrogate our own readings of these data. As importantly, these quotes also serve to forcefully illustrate (in a way paraphrasing cannot) the technical, social, ethical and practical complexities with which practitioners within the HIV prevention field struggle.

Chapter 7, the concluding chapter, begins by summarizing our key observations and distilling our general analytic perspective as we have elaborated it over the course of the book. We then draw out some of the implications of this for the analysis of the HIV field more broadly, and outline the ways in which this approach might illuminate the relations between biomedicine and innovation in general. However, we also begin to address what it would mean practically to take seriously the prospective dimensions, or 'virtuality', of events. If events are open, or have the possibility of being open, are there ways in which this openness can be proactively encouraged? As such, we sketch out some ideas about how this might take place. In particular, we draw on the methodology and ontology of 'speculative design' as a means of practically interjecting in PrEP RCTs such that they are not simply occasions in which solutions are sought for pre-specified problems, but events in which inventive problem-making can emerge, problem-making that better and more usefully accommodates the complexities of PrEP, its potential users and its trials.

2
A Brief and Partial History of Randomized Controlled Trials (RCTs) in the Context of HIV Prevention and Treatment

Introduction

In this chapter we provide a partial history of randomized controlled trials (RCTs) as they have been applied within the HIV field in pursuit of prevention technologies. These RCTs are mostly prior to pre-exposure prophylactics (PrEP) and the account presented here is meant to contextualize our main object of study, PrEP, and particularly the controversies that surrounded the first round of PrEP RCTs. Central to the story of the early PrEP trials as told by various interested parties (for example, activists, trialists) was the question of whether these trials were devised in what amounts to an unethical manner. Also at stake in these debates was whether these concerns could be equally applied to other HIV prevention trials. As we shall see, some actors have been adamant that the PrEP trials in which they were involved were ethical; others have maintained that the requirements to inform and protect participants were not met; and a third group have questioned why the early PrEP trials provoked controversy when, in their view, issues of protecting participants were not so different to other prevention trials. Informing all three positions are some key assumptions that underpin the rationale for clinical trials – a rationale in which RCTs come to be regarded as the 'gold standard' for achieving evidence-based research within the HIV field. Part and parcel of this is the institution and institutionalization of particular ethical standards. Within the HIV biomedical prevention field, as with many other areas of clinical research, science and ethics (or, more specifically, bioethics) are enacted as if distinct endeavours, informed by the two disciplinary approaches of the natural sciences and moral philosophy. In this chapter we will begin to suggest that this separation serves to legitimate a particular form of evidence gathering that restricts what can be understood by the challenge of the HIV epidemic. This chapter thus sets out, in a series of historical vignettes, the ways in which this relation between trials and ethics acts to constrain the sorts of questions that can be asked about HIV prevention. However, as a proviso on the coming discussion, we should state that we have resisted articulating our own analytic view on bioethics in this chapter. We deal more fully with the literature on bioethics in Chapter 3. Here, we are primarily interested in exemplifying how bioethics is operationalized and implemented in the HIV field. One advantage of this tack is that we can subsequently draw on these empirical examples in order to interrogate the bioethics literature.

In what follows, we will provide a wide range of empirical examples of trials that have tested particular interventions in the HIV field. Our aim is to demonstrate in broad strokes how these trials systematically bracket a range of factors that, both ethically and epistemologically, might prove highly pertinent. Of particular significance is that our argument corresponds, in some respects, with the concerns of those centrally involved in implementing and upholding the presumed 'gold standard' evidence-based research technology of the RCT (see, for example, Padian et al., 2010). As we show through our examples of the problematic nature of a number of RCTs, frequently those involved recognize and struggle with the limitations of their data. It is this commitment to the technology of the RCT, and the simultaneous recognition that its capacity to deal concretely with HIV transmissions is highly problematic, that has inspired us. Indeed, it is this conundrum that has led us to propose that a more valuable form of evidence to be derived from the RCT rests on a more open-ended engagement with the dynamic and highly relational nature of HIV. In this sense, the chapter also serves as an empirical backdrop to the conceptual discussion in Chapter 3 where we develop an analytic framework for addressing just these elements of open-endedness, dynamism and relationality (as well as a few others).

Some early problems with HIV RCTs

From early on in the epidemic, trials – although not always involving randomization – have been the main technology for devising HIV treatment and prevention interventions. They have also been the subject of contention, although – as each involves different 'stuff', for example, different foci, bodies, drugs, measures, locales – the concerns raised by their practice have differed. Steven Epstein's (1996) account of the epidemic up until the advent of effective antiretroviral combination therapy, *Impure Science*, opens with a description of public protest by the Boston chapter of the activist group ACT UP (the AIDS Coalition to Unleash Power) demanding 'an end to medical elitism and "elegant science"' (1996:1,2). In this instance, ACT UP queried the purpose of trialling the single drug AZT that was already known to, on the one hand, display high toxicity and, on the other, have limited effect on viral suppression. The protest demands were, Epstein suggested, emblematic of the intense engagement with science by those affected by the virus. It was an engagement that served to complexify any simple view of the purity of science; crucially, it was this 'impurity' (albeit one that inevitably reflected the cultural ideas of its time), that was directed foremost toward the benefit of those for whom science ostensibly labours, namely, those infected with, or at high risk of, HIV. In effect, then, questions about the ethicality of science were in place from the outset of the epidemic. Similarly, and particularly pertinent to what we discuss in relation to the PrEP trials, in Cindy Patton's writing (1990:59) about the early days of the epidemic and the initial naming of AIDS as GRID (gay-related immune deficiency), we find an account of what she characterized as the hegemonic nature of science in its framing of HIV risk. As she phrased it, the ability of science to arbitrate on true or correct knowledge had the effect of excluding community knowledge and, hence, precisely that knowledge necessary for 'transmission interruption' (Patton, 1990:54). Patton was referring primarily to the situation in the United States and the manner in which medical science viewed the virus through the prism of a version of identity politics in which desire for same sex was conflated with the disease. Accordingly, this emphasis neglected the crucial role of risky *practices* and the complex relations that these entailed.

In our discussion of current RCTs of PrEP, we will suggest that parallel, if somewhat substantively different, patterns of inclusion and exclusion have been in operation. As the epidemic has extended to some of the most impoverished areas of the world *and* has become more medicalized with the success of combination antiretroviral drug treatments for viral suppression in those infected (hereon referred to as seropositive), the nature of the contentiousness of RCTs has altered. In place of the activism witnessed in what is often referred to as the 'global north' of the epidemic – for example, the United States, Canada, Western Europe and, although geographically South, Australia – the most predominant voices are now those of international organizations, government agencies and biomedical scientists advocating solutions to the growing infection rates and poor treatment access in Southern Africa, Asia, Eastern Europe and parts of South America. In place of lay challenges to medical elitism and 'elegant science' (Epstein, 1996:1,2), a new set of biomedically oriented actors have emerged to lead a different sort of struggle. It is a struggle to spread the word and practice of science. The RCT, itself, has become a more widespread and virtually *unquestioned* mode of evidence gathering (for a discussion on this topic, see, for example, Kippax et al., 2011; Kippax and Holt, 2009; Mykhalovskiy and Rosengarten, 2009; Mykhalovskiy and Weir, 2004) and, in light of this, a primary goal has become one of securing the participation of individual members of HIV vulnerable communities *in* it (UNAIDS/AVAC, 2011).

However, it is as a consequence of securing highly vulnerable individuals in RCTs that those who have embraced this so-called 'gold standard' technology, on occasion, find themselves under fire for the ethicality of their commitment to and implementation of RCTs. Our interest is in how concern about ethicality is framed, notably how it serves to give legitimacy to what, in effect, is a costly – financially but also in human resource terms – process which, despite its celebrated 'gold standard' status, frames solutions that are, in fact, often not workable. That is to say, a consistent neglect of the reductive tendencies of science and the effects of this on the expressed goal of HIV prevention suggests that it has become imperative to reframe the problem.

RCTs and what they can exclude

The RCT (an abbreviation that sometimes stands for randomized controlled trial and sometimes for randomized clinical trial) is now accepted as the most effective method for testing drug safety (Phase I trials) before extending to efficacy testing (Phase II/III).[1] Indeed, its popularity is now so pronounced that it is used to assess social interventions in HIV (see, for example, Stephenson et al., 2003). Here it will be discussed in terms of its role in the resilience of HIV biomedical research in spite of a range of challenges. All phases of RCTs have control arms for comparative purposes: the same or a similar number of research subjects to those receiving the trial candidate are allocated to a group that receives a placebo or a product whose efficacy has already been established. The process of randomization is usually carried out in a manner that matches certain characteristics across the arms, for example, an RCT that intentionally studies men who have sex with men (MSM) and transgender people will randomize the research subjects to ensure that a near-equal number of these identity categories are represented in the different arms. Statistical measures are used to establish whether differences in anticipated outcomes between the two or more arms – in the case of HIV prevention RCTs the differences would pertain to HIV infections – are evidence of the product's efficacy. The 'offshore' RCT – HIV-directed or otherwise – which we discuss below, is typically situated in sites at some distance from the trial sponsor's country or region of origin: usually, at these offshore locations health and medical services and support are significantly less available (MacQueen et al., 2007).

Beyond the HIV biomedical field, the RCT has become an increasingly legitimized experimental tool for testing pharmaceutical drugs, not least when that testing is conducted 'offshore'. According to Adriana Petryna in her studies of the research and development practices of large pharmaceutical companies (2005, 2007), 'offshore' RCTs are able to recruit high numbers of trial participants because they offer a health and/or medical intervention otherwise locally unavailable. The need for the intervention therefore increases the likelihood that the RCT will gain approval from the government of a low or middle-income country. However, reliance on a pharmaceutical industry RCT for provision of a needed health or medical intervention leaves public health systems vulnerable to market motivated interests. The corporate trial sponsor may withdraw at a 'whim' if the relevant government, or indeed other factors, impede their commercial interests (Petryna, 2007:35). Interest in the use of offshore locales for testing new drugs outside the HIV field derives from the lower monetary cost of running an RCT in a country poorer than that of the trial sponsor and in which there is availability of significantly high numbers of people suitable for testing.

These features are characteristic of HIV 'offshore' RCTs in part only. Although the undertaking of the 'offshore' trials is common in order to achieve high numbers of people suitable for testing, and although asymmetries in resource provisions are especially apparent, most HIV RCTs are not controlled by the pharmaceutical industry. Rather, they are the result of an intricate relationship between the trial sponsor, the trialists, the national public health authority and the affected community. There is often a direct exchange of expertise between bench scientists employed by the pharmaceutical company and trialists employed by a university. Indeed, funding may come from the pharmaceutical industry and/or a philanthropic or public organization and it is not easy to disentangle the contributions of different sectors. Possibly the difficulty of doing so tells us something of how the HIV prevention field itself involves intricate synergistic relations amongst actors who elsewhere may be assumed to pursue different, even competing, interests in relation to private/corporate funded and public research. As the anthropologist Denielle Elliot (2011) explains:

> While many may see the absence of industry from AIDS prevention research as auspicious, it does not account for the entanglements between industry, states, universities and the market...Nor does it account for the political and economic influence that new NGOs, like the Gates Foundation or Family Health International, wield in the global AIDS and humanitarian industries.

Even without a clear account of market motivation or, to put this in more commonplace terms, commodity greed, this does not necessarily immunize those organizing HIV RCTs from the sort of criticism levelled some time ago at biomedicine by Patton that we noted above. The arrangements between the different actors mentioned by Elliot have become manifest in the support now available for large funding programmes for bench science and RCTs. As MacQueen (2011) notes, there remains comparatively little focus on social scientific research. Mostly what is available is restricted to behavioural surveillance studies seeking to determine, for example, rates of unprotected sex (coitus without a condom) or rates of dosing adherence. Further, it can be noted that more 'classical' interventions such as integrated condom programmes have received less backing or study – perhaps unsurprising in light of Kippax's (2003) observation that the effectiveness of the male condom has generally been undersold amongst those associated with the deployment of RCTs in the HIV field. Although a number of social scientists repeatedly seek to remind their biomedical colleagues that HIV transmission takes place through sex and injecting drug use, that is, through practices that are profoundly social, and thus that any biomedical technology will be affected by social relations in its take up (Auerbach and Coates, 2000; Auerbach et al., 2011; Kippax and Holt, 2009; Kippax and Stephenson, 2012), this appears to be largely ignored. Nguyen et al. (2011:291) go so far as to argue that expressions of triumphalism about recent trial results for PrEP (and for other uses of antiretroviral drugs for prevention of sexual transmission) imply that integrated condom programmes do not work. This neglect persists despite what Nguyen et al. (2011) note as crucial evidence, of late, that such programmes have resulted in the declining incidence of HIV infection in youth in the most affected countries.

In order to provide an overview of resource allocation toward prevention measures, Peters et al. (2010) offer an analysis of the financial resource flows from the US and Europe for integrated condom programming (non-biomedical) and for vaccine and microbicide (a substance for surface vaginal or anal protection or an oral pill) research (including oral PrEP). They conclude 'there is a remarkable shift away from supporting low cost and effective technologies [the male condom] to funding research into as of yet not proven high technology HIV preventives' (2010:13). That this shift occurs despite lack of evidence is especially worrying and lends still more support to Patton's (1990:54) account of the 'hegemonic' status of the logic and methods of the biological sciences in the early stages of the epidemic. It is difficult to avoid the nagging question arising from Peters et al.'s (2010) analysis: why is there so much support for little proven or, in the case of PrEP, highly challenging technologies, when it is well established that condoms are the cheapest, safest and most effective means of preventing transmission?

According to one set of biomedical scientists (see below; Padian et al., 2008), it seems that a particular notion of urgency has justified the singular investment in 'a biological fix', leading one to wonder if the promise of science has an allure that overshadows more complex, less exotic or 'innovatory' engagements that might better achieve prevention (such as the distribution of condoms).

We glimpse this justification for the combination of biological fix and RCT in the following brief statement from Padian et al. (2008:586):

> One of the early success stories [in the history of the epidemic] was the increased use of condoms in high-risk locations, such as bath houses in the USA and brothels in Thailand; increased use of male condoms had a measurable effect on reduction of HIV transmission in these contexts. Simultaneously, HIV was seen to be spreading at a devastating pace in sub-Saharan Africa and the primary means of transmission was through heterosexual intercourse. Changes in sexual behaviour that had occurred in selected communities at risk of HIV infection were too small and too slow to bring this new epidemic quickly under control. Thus, the search for a quick technological, biological fix that did not rely on behaviour began in earnest.

Unfortunately there has been no speedy 'biological fix,' and nearly three decades have passed during which the only evidence-based 'biological fix' has been the use of antiretroviral drugs in the prevention of mother-to-child transmission (PMTC). Indeed, other than a long lasting one-off highly efficacious vaccine, it is hard to imagine what such a fix might be. As Kippax and Stephenson (2012:789) explain, all HIV prevention interventions 'including those that are called biomedical, must engage with the lived world of those at risk for infection'. By ignoring what has worked, Padian et al. (2008) foreclose on what else might be achieved without drug interventions.

However, our key point at this stage in our discussion is that the problematic nature of PrEP can be reframed in a more productive way better to serve prevention efforts. Our argument is that the problem of PrEP, now faced by public health officials and others, might well have emerged differently had a less bifurcated enactment of the epidemic been possible, one which avoided the distinction between 'biomedical' and 'social' interventions.[2]

Padian et al.'s (2008) account of how biomedical approaches acquired their pre-eminence is entirely consistent with a methodological perspective in which RCTs pursue measures of 'efficacy' as a necessary precursor to measures of 'effectiveness'. Thus, the essence of a biomedical technology must first be revealed prior to considering the relationship of that technology to 'uncontrolled' conditions such as the limits to participant access, or shifting gender relations, and changing local conceptions of risk (Kippax and Stephenson, 2012). This is further evidenced in another statement from Padian et al. (2008:593), which again privileges 'efficacy' results: 'If adequate adherence is not achieved [by the user of a topical microbicide or oral PrEP] during a study, *the true prevention* [our emphasis] effect will be masked.' Here we begin to see the performative work of the 'biological fix': the 'fix' comes into view as that which will follow from the work of the RCT even while it is already at work in affording the RCT its validity. In other words, there is a circular logic at play here. It is the expectation that the RCT will deliver – and, moreover, deliver what is necessary while bracketing many of the conditions under which the intervention might actually work – that we wish to bring into the foreground. Moreover, within this circular logic, there is a structure of expectation (we expand on expectations in Chapter 3) that incorporates a particular version of bioethics that likewise contributes to the shaping of what comes to be seen as the 'key' prevention intervention, that is, the 'biological fix'.

In the next section we review the way in which a series of RCTs have been undertaken in pursuit of an 'efficacious' intervention. In addition to RCTs that have been conducted to develop, variously, a topical microbicide and a vaccine against HIV, we also draw attention to an emerging issue concerning dubious proposals for HIV eradication following evidence that viral suppression in seropositive people reduces risk of transmission.

More trials, more exclusions...

We begin with a discussion of efforts to develop topical microbicides (for vaginal or anal surface protection) and how, despite having emerged from a political campaign to meet the needs of users, these efforts exemplify what we noted above as a bracketing of factors that can be linked to a longstanding lack of success. The sort of user needs that the Global Campaign for Microbicides (GCM) sought to incorporate in the design of their topical microbicides resulted in the idea that a number of different microbicides would be necessary. For it was soon recognized that a microbicide would need to: provide contraception as well as protection against HIV; provide protection from HIV but still allow conception; provide protection for anal intercourse recognizing the needs of both women and men; enable insertion prior to coitus without affecting the pleasure of intercourse as a result of over-lubrication from a gel, cream or suppository; and not be materially detectable to a sexual partner.[3]

The political campaign and the sort of user needs noted above reflected what can be characterized as the concerns of a women's health movement. That is to say, advocates who saw themselves working for vulnerable women and not necessarily with the intent of prioritizing scientific logic, enlisted science to help redress the situation of women. To some extent this has also informed a critique of RCTs. One of the most significant initiators, and a continued supporter, of the campaign for topical microbicides is the prominent epidemiologist, Zena Stein. In 1990, Stein problematized the distinction between a scientific concern with 'efficacy' over 'effectiveness,' pointing out that a reliance on 'efficacy' measures of condoms – showing that they statistically protected against HIV infection – was irrelevant if women were unable to use condoms in practice. The claim underscored the importance of a female-initiated intervention:

> In the more developed world and the less developed world, a key problem with the condom from the point of view of the woman is that it calls upon the woman to assert dominance in the sexual act. Almost everywhere such dominance is not the traditional mode, and imposes unfamiliar behaviour on both members of the couple. Logic dictates that the educational message about condoms, to be effective, must be targeted at the man or couple. If targeted at the woman, she

in turn has to persuade her partner, and therein lays the difficulty. (Stein 1990:2 in Van der Zaag, unpublished)

The microbicide initiatives have clearly taken these lessons to heart. However, as we shall see, this did not avert what eventually turned out to be a fraught history. Indeed, according to Van der Zaag (unpublished), the project of seeking to 'empower women' who are otherwise sexually and economically subordinate to men by providing them with a prevention technology that they can use – with or without 'his' knowledge – now raises questions about whether the marriage of advocacy and science has generated its own susceptibilities.

It was only in 2010 that the first positive results by the CAPRISA topical microbicide trial were released. Although the results indicated 'proof of concept' (Van Damme and Szpir, 2012:520) and not efficacy (that is, evidence to show the product works but not on a basis sufficient to generalize to a population) – Stein's challenge to the efficacy/effectiveness distinction notwithstanding – they generated much excitement.[4] The CAPRISA trial tested Tenofovir Gel (an intervention using one of the drugs in oral PrEP) and is reported to have achieved 39 percent reduction in risk (Abdool Karim, 2010:1172). These results came after a battery of relatively unsuccessful trials. One of these was the especially disturbing finding by the nonoxynol9 RCT that the product resulted in harm to the research subjects.

Between 1996 and 2000, the nonoxynol9 RCT, which went by the study name of COL-1492, was conducted with 892 female sex workers in four countries: Benin, Côte d'Ivoire, South Africa and Thailand. Approximately half of the participants were asked to insert the vaginal spermicide nonoxynol-9. The rationale for the nonoxynol-9 RCT drew on the existing availability of nonoxynol-9 already licensed for use as a contraceptive and suggestions that it might offer some protection against HIV. Unexpectedly, in place of a demonstrated protective effect, the RCT found that multiple use of nonoxynol-9 caused toxic effects that actually enabled HIV-1 infection (Van Damme et al., 2002). In other words, the spermicide increased some women's susceptibility to HIV infection.

Other HIV biomedical prevention RCTs for a topical microbicide have been more innocuous in their findings, and have been recorded simply as achieving no significant results to suggest protective effect. So, in spite of the more promising outcomes of the CAPRISA trial, it is apparent from this brief historical sketch that many years of research to develop a topical microbicide have achieved relatively little for HIV prevention.

In part, we suggest, that the poor outcomes of prevention RCTs follow from a framing that constitutes an 'intervention' and a 'user' as distinct and stable entities and, as such, cannot conceive of how these act on and effect what each become. Reviewing the outcome of the nonoxynol-9 trial, it seems appropriate to deduce that what functioned as a 'spermicide', that is, an agent intended to disable sperm in order to prevent pregnancy from penis/vagina coitus became a different kind of toxic substance when HIV was present. That is to say, the entities of sperm, vagina, spermicide and HIV affected the material properties of each in a manner different to when HIV was not present. In more succinct terms, in association with HIV the spermicide acquired a different materiality that left the female body susceptible to infection.

In the following statement we see another example of how an explanatory frame of distinct stable entities leaves trialists struggling to make sense of data, in this instance a gel and coitus. The investigators for the CAPRISA RCT state:

> In this study [CAPRISA] population, women with the highest gel adherence tended to have the lowest reported coital frequency. Despite their lower coital frequency, these women had HIV incidence rates comparable (in the placebo gel arm) with those women with much higher coital frequencies, highlighting the importance of infrequent but very high-risk sex with migrant men. The impact of coitally related tenofovir gel was substantial in this group, indicating its potential to alter the course of the HIV epidemic in southern Africa, where young women engaging in sex with migrant men is the key driver in the spread of HIV infection. On a cautionary note, the effectiveness of coitally related tenofovir gel appeared to decline after 18 months; reasons for this are unclear, and factors, including the possibility of declining number of gel applications and/or adherence over time, need further investigation. (Abdool Karim et al., 2010:1172, 1173)

The 'cautionary note' serves to occlude from consideration a more dynamic relationality at work in HIV prevention. Indeed despite copious evidence that conceptions of HIV risk and prevention practices alter with time and in relation to various phenomena (see, for example, Cassell et al., 2006; Rosengarten, 2009), the explanatory frame remains tied to the possibility of a 'pure' gel (topical microbicide) that can be studied apart from the practice of its use.

Even before efforts to develop a topical microbicide, researchers began to pursue an HIV vaccine.[5] A vaccine has long been regarded as the preferred prevention technology, not only because of its possible effectiveness for preventing transmission but also because it might offer a means of curing HIV or reducing the destructive capacity of the virus. Importantly vaccines are not tied to coitus and, in light of the success of smallpox and polio vaccines, can be assumed to be both non-toxic and stimulators of an immune response (itself imagined as essentially positive). But as we discuss below, and not unlike the story of topical microbicides, the development of an HIV vaccine has also been immensely disappointing and largely fraught, with only recent success.

In 2010, the biggest RCT ever undertaken to date, ALVAC-AIDSVAX (RV 144), showed that vaccine recipients were 31 per cent less likely than placebo recipients to become HIV-infected. The RCT recruited 16,402 Thai adults aged between 18 and 30. However, at the time of writing, the biological mechanism responsible for this effective protection has not been isolated (Grant and Bass, 2010).[6] Prior to this 'proof of concept,' in the words of the International AIDS Vaccine Initiative (IAVI) which co-ordinates the HIV vaccine trials network, 'dozens of studies to advance the development of safe and effective AIDS vaccines' have been carried out (IAVI, 2012). Although most of these trials have been recorded as having no deleterious effect, another more recent study, the STEP trial, bore some resonance to the above mentioned nonoxynol-9 microbicide trial. Contrary to its aim of, if not preventing infection outright, possibly reducing the effects of infection, it increased the HIV vulnerability of some of its research subjects.[7] The study demonstrated that the vaccine did not prevent infection, nor did it lower the viral load in those who became infected. But the results also showed that some groups of men who received the vaccine (namely, those who had antibodies to a common cold, were uncircumcised and received a planned repeat vaccination) may have been, and may continue to be, more likely to become infected when exposed to the virus than those who received the placebo. Again we encounter the sheer complexity of what goes into an RCT (circumcision, having a cold, double vaccination) – what we shall later refer to as its eventuation – and the fraught outcomes that follow in the wake of this complexity. To reiterate, the point is that a version of the RCT that is effectively exclusionary can be counterposed to a version of the RCT that is more encompassing of, and adaptable to, these emerging exigencies.

The tendency to exclude complexity is especially apparent in the way findings of recent 'successful' trials have been, and continue to be, taken up as part of what some argue is the worrisome biomedicalization of prevention (Nguyen 2011; Kippax and Holt, 2009). Most notable is the manner in which the findings of male circumcision RCTs have led to the funding and implementation of programmes for widespread circumcision of adult men in some sub-Saharan African countries (WHO,

2012a). In spite of various concerns raised (see, for example, Dowsett and Couch, 2007), there appears to be no follow-up social research on the implications of this intervention for those who undergo it, nor studies of whether other prevention practices – especially the use of the male condom – are sustained. However, it is the claims for 'treatment as prevention' (TasP) that have generated the most debate. Findings from the TasP HPTN052 on the effect of viral suppression by antiretrovirals to prevent HIV transmission within serodiscordant heterosexual regular relationships (Lancet, 2011) have resulted in calls for early intervention with antiretroviral therapy, even before these have been clinically recommended (Montaner et al., 2006; Eaten et al., 2012) along with claims that an end to the epidemic is in sight. Yet many in the field argue that a more complex analysis of how this strategy will work – politically, ethically, medically, economically and in terms of actually significantly reducing HIV infections – is of critical importance (Adam, 2011; Nguyen et al., 2011; Barnighausen et al., 2012; Holtgrave et al., 2012). According to Smith et al. (2012), there are several limitations with the RCT itself, namely that assumptions are made about the effects of drugs which are based on generating data that does not necessarily reflect what happens at the individual level or in specific contexts. For instance, although antiretrovirals can be demonstrated to reduce infectivity, this effect cannot be assumed to take place in actuality. For Smith et al. (2012:2) it is possible that some people who are diagnosed as HIV positive will be lost to follow up and, hence, to treatment take up. As a result, their infectivity will not be reduced. The same authors note that people with acute infection may pass on the virus before being diagnosed and these individuals may contribute disproportionally toward onward transmission (2012:2). They further note that diagnoses of HIV infection – central to the effectiveness of this intervention – will be affected by changes in the availability of services and individual testing behaviours (2012:4).

To summarize this section, we have examined how a number of interventions have been tested, and noted that the use of RCTs in such testing, with their typical bracketing of the sociomaterial complexities entailed in the use of those interventions, have been generative of a series of highly problematic issues.

Offshore trials and further complexities

In this section we review some of the complex ways in which the off-shore-ness of RCTs has been played out in terms of bioethics. In part this involves describing some of the more contentious RCTs that have attracted widespread attention but this also allows us to reflect on how ethics has been, and continues to be, enacted. All the RCTs mentioned above have been 'offshore' or have included offshore locations containing the majority of participants. Bearing in mind that participating in an RCT involves some risk if the product candidate produces unexpected effects, it is possible to say already that those in poorer settings with fewer health and medical resources available to them have been, and continue to be, at greater risk than participants of RCTs based in the RCT's 'home' country where 'state-of-the-art' medicine is available. As MacQueen et al. (2007:554) explain:

> Epidemiologically, they [people in developing countries] are the people with the greatest need for effective prevention; statistically, they also present the most efficient opportunity to test interventions but the poverty and disempowerment that generate vulnerability to HIV infection also serve as barriers to medical care and services. Thus, the people most appropriate for enrolment [sic] in international HIV prevention trials are also the people least likely to have access to HIV treatment and care in their local communities.

Following MacQueen et al. (2007), we can say from the outset of our discussion that the 'offshore-ness' of HIV RCTs bare a type of inbuilt ethical dilemma. In turn, this raises questions about the way in which such trials locate themselves in relation to local resources. Although it is increasingly the case that such trials involve local scientific researchers and engage in explicit capacity building, there remains a tension between the state of the art medical benefits that inform their practice and the quality of the local surrounding health and medical facilities. To put this another way, while the RCT has been able to travel and exploit the effects of local conditions that generate high numbers of people vulnerable to HIV, the relationship has not always been reciprocal. RCTs have remained largely immune from expectations that they 'share their resources'. In some previous instances, the asymmetries between the home of the trial sponsor and the trial location in a low or middle-income country have been handled so brazenly that they have attracted the critical attention of medical and ethics professionals beyond the HIV field. Below we provide a rather lengthy discussion of two particular RCTs to show how asymmetries in resources are inscribed in and hence re-enacted by the design of RCTs. We also signal the manner in which ethics has been framed as part of a broad consternation about these RCTs, noting that the nature of the framing leaves the question of what is ethical open to debate and, for some, subject to disqualification.

Our first example is a RCT carried out in Uganda between 1994 and 1998 with the aim of studying the influence of viral load on heterosexual transmission of HIV in relation to such risk factors as sexually transmitted infections (STIs) including gonorrhoea and syphilis. This RCT has been adjudged unethical because it unnecessarily involved deliberately leaving people untreated (although they were told treatment could be obtained elsewhere); this would not have been found acceptable in the country of the sponsor. The RCT recruited residents from ten villages without access to antiretroviral treatment and identified 415 couples in which one partner was HIV positive and one was initially HIV negative and followed them prospectively for up to 30 months. During this period, residents of five of the villages were treated for sexually transmitted infections (excluding HIV) and compared to residents in the other villages who were not treated when an infection was identified (those untreated were referred to free government clinics).

The RCT was unable to find that STIs affected the transmission of HIV but did find that increased viral load was a significant factor for transmission risk.

In a review of this study, Marcia Angell, editor of the *New England of Journal of Medicine* raised questions about the futility of the trial given evidence that showed that an increased viral load – already demonstrated at that time to be susceptible to suppression by antiretroviral therapy – was associated with a greater risk of transmission. But, even leaving aside this latter issue and the absence of access to AIDS-preventing antiretroviral drugs for those who were seropositive, Angell (2000:967) was still able to claim: 'Such a study could not have been performed in the United States, where it would be expected that patients with HIV and other sexually transmitted diseases would be treated.'

In short, that the history of HIV prevention trials is fraught, we suggest, has much to do with how the trials themselves can be defended against what are in effect a set of universalized principles (that is, the provision of treatment for infections such as STDs). Although Angell's argument draws attention to how locally specific conditions of poverty appear to have generated practices that not only reflected global asymmetries but effectively reproduced them, the trial itself can nevertheless be warranted as causing no harm. Such an argument depends, of course, on what is understood as harm, a point we develop taking into account our next example.

The second RCT we want to mention also attracted critical comment from beyond the field (see, for example, de Zulueta, 2001; Lurie and Wolfe, 1997). It compared the use of the antiretroviral drug AZT (zidovudine) with a placebo and was designed to test AZT's capacity for preventing mother to child transmission in southern Africa. The trial followed the Protocol 076 trial which had been conducted in the US and was so successful in its results that it was stopped early on the grounds that it would be unethical to continue the placebo arm. However, the intervention provided by Protocol 076 trial in the US was regarded as too complex and, therefore, not feasible for delivery in southern Africa.[8] On the basis that a simpler intervention might work, a shorter course of the drug was offered and compared with a placebo. That is to say, although there was already strong evidence of an efficacious intervention, the trial was designed with a placebo arm. The placebo arm was claimed to be justified on the grounds that it was equivalent to the conditions that the research subjects would otherwise experience in their local contexts (Ho, 1997:83 cited by Craddock, 2004:243). But in effect this meant that the design of the RCT unnecessarily involved children born to mothers in the placebo arm acquiring preventable HIV. Another way of putting this is that the epidemic and recognized local specificities, together, generated a new technical design but also, a particular account of what is ethical. Potentially preventable infections were deemed acceptable because they were differentiated by a particular account of local specificity.

In place of accepting the assertion of particular sorts of differences and notionally indicating that ethics resides in how a context is enacted, Lurie and Wolfe (1997) propose that a different research question would have avoided the ethical compromise evident in the AZT RCTs. In place of comparing a reduced intervention (the experimental arm) with no intervention (as was the current context), which would certainly leave women in the no intervention/placebo arm very likely to give birth to children with otherwise preventable HIV infection, they proposed the placebo arm be replaced with the US-demonstrated prevention vention. In their view, the ethical and research effective question would have been: 'Can we reduce the duration of prophylactic [zidovudine] treatment [the experimental option] without increasing the risk of perinatal transmission of HIV, that is, without compromising the demonstrated efficacy of the standard ACTG 076 [zidovudine] regimen? [shown efficacious in the US]' (1997:854). The reformulation of the research design posed in Lurie and Wolfe's question meant that instead of half of the women being randomly assigned to the no intervention arm, all the women in the southern African trials would be given accarm, all the women in the southern African trials would have been given access to some form of prevention: in this way, it would still have been possible to assess the efficacy of the experimental intervention.

Less frequently considered within the HIV field, but evoked by MacQueen et al.'s (2007) commentary, are trial-incurred health and medical needs of individual participants that, in turn, may engender new demands on already inadequate familial, local and national resources at offshore sites. This can be seen with RCTs that produce unanticipated adverse events over the course of their duration, for instance, the STEP vaccine trial discussed above. But further, adverse events do not always manifest within the timeframe of a trial. They can develop long after the trialists have left the site and diagnostic health follow up has ceased. Amongst these (and one that can be regarded as a 'social' adverse event) is the well-articulated concern that HIV prevention RCTs may give people a false sense of the risk of HIV and discourage or 'inhibit' safe sex practices with long term effects (Cassell et al., 2006).

What is ethics when it relies *on* HIV infections in order to prevent them?

One of the features, to date, of the HIV biomedical prevention RCT that leads it to seek out 'offshore' locales has been the technical requirement that participants, in at least the placebo arm, can become HIV infected in order to demonstrate that participants in both arms have been exposed to the virus. Exposure is the means of establishing whether the intervention offers protection (Bass and Kahn, 2005). And it is the feature of people becoming infected during their enrolment in the trial – termed 'intercurrent infection' – that has generated most consternation and some debate.

Until recently there was no obligation on trialists to provide antiretroviral treatment for 'intercurrent infection'. The ethical justification for this continues to rest on the view that intercurrent infection is not a result of the trial but of the participant's own unsafe activities (Haire, 2011). One of the counter arguments put forward seeks to shift the frame from the liberal notion of a possessive individual responsible for his or her own behaviour to a structural one where the conditions – such as lack of other sources of income that make sex work necessary – that justify the offshore location of the trial are precisely those that give rise to HIV infection. In direct contrast to the published position of UNAIDS/WHO (2007), this view claims that trialists have an obligation to treat intercurrent HIV infection because it arises not as a result of individual failure but *due to the same conditions integral to the trial* (Haire, 2011), that is, those conditions that render the offshore location attractive to the trialists in the first place. Indeed, on the basis of this viewpoint, it would seem that in conditions where there is an absence of sufficient healthcare infrastructure – which facilitates the risk of infection – the ethical obligation on trialists becomes all the greater.

There is an unsettling irony in the occurrence of HIV infection as it is precisely what the researchers have declared themselves against – the awfulness of HIV infection – in seeking to devise a prevention technology. Hence many researchers are now committing to the future provision of ARVs for those who become HIV infected during the trial (Kahn, 2005). However, we cannot help but note that the increasing commitment to providing care for those who do become infected arises in a changing historical context. It coincides with the expansion of antiretroviral access that makes this provision feasible, whereas an earlier commitment would have placed the feasibility of the trial in question. It is the last point that requires something more than the structural critique outlined above.

By continuing to locate intercurrent infection as 'other' to the RCT, that is, outside the trial and due to either 'bad' behaviour or lack of institutional support, the complex network of relations inherent to the operations of the trial are overlooked. It is through these operations that a number of claims and failed promises are enabled. Intercurrent infection, as one example, acquires its meaning as such in relation to the trial and, more critically, the trial is only able to draw meaningful results through its occurrence. That is to say, intercurrent infection cannot be sustained as 'outside' the workings of the trial. Rather HIV infections are an in-built feature of the current design of the HIV biomedical prevention RCT. In the terms we shall develop in the next chapter, intercurrent infections are key elements in what we shall call the 'eventuation' of a trial, where eventuation signals, amongst other things, the widening of what can be included as a constituent part of a trial. Over the course of our discussion of PrEP below, we will come back to many of the questions raised in the foregoing.

PrEP trials: From inauspicious beginnings to mighty challenges

It is in light of the problematic manner in which RCTs can be understood to take place, that we now review the findings and challenges of recent PrEP trials. To date, four large PrEP RCTs have been undertaken and their results released as follows:

1. The iPrEX trial which tested the efficacy of once-daily TDF/FTC (brand name Truvada) in 2,499 gay men, transgender women and other men who have sex with men at sites in six countries – Brazil, Ecuador, Peru, South Africa, Thailand and the US. The results, released in November 2010, found Truvada reduced risk of HIV infection by an average of 44 per cent. A significantly higher percentage of protection (92 per cent) was found in those with high dosing adherence (Grant et al., 2010).
2. The Partners PrEP study in Kenya and Uganda enrolled 4,758 heterosexual couples in which one partner was seropositive and the other seronegative. In the trial, daily oral TDF (Tenofovir on its own) reduced HIV risk by an estimated 62 per cent infections and daily oral TDF/FTC (Tenofovir combined with Emtricitabine and called Truvada) reduced HIV risk by an estimated 73 per cent when compared to a placebo. Both drugs were effective in both men and women (Baeten et al. 2012).
3. The TDF2 study in Botswana enrolled just over 1,200 sexually active men and women. Although not designed to assess efficacy (expanded safety only), analysis of final data on numbers of infections in the active and placebo arms indicated that daily oral TDF/FTC (Truvada) reduced the risk of HIV infection in both men and women participants by an estimated 62.6 per cent compared to those who received the placebo (Thigpen et al., 2012).
4. In April 2011, the FEM-PrEP study was discontinued after seeking to test the same drugs and daily dosage of TDF/FTC (Truvada) as above in 2000 women. The decision to stop the trial was made by the Independent Data Monitoring Committee (IDMC) due to ongoing lack of statistical differences between the product and placebo arms of the trial (Van Damme et al., 2012)

At the time of writing, two trials are in process:

1. CDC 4370: Study of the Safety and Efficacy of Daily Tenofovir-Disoproxil Fumarate (TDF) to Prevent HIV Infection among Injection Drug Users (2,400 injecting drug users) in Bangkok, Thailand. It is arguably the most contentious trial of all those planned and/or undertaken and still subject to the considerations raised in 2005 as we discuss below. (AVAC, 2013)
2. VOICE (MTN-003) comparing safety and efficacy of both oral and topical uses of the antiretroviral compounds and single and dual drugs in oral form (TDF and TDF/FTC) in 5,000 women in Malawi, South

Africa, Uganda and Zimbabwe whose primary risk factor is vaginal sex. Results, to date, are uneven and as we discuss in Chapter 4 perplexing for the trialists. Whereas Tenofovir (single drug version of PrEP) was found to be efficacious in women as well as in men in the Partners study (cited above), the lack of results in the arm of VOICE trialling the same pill (in pharmaceutical terms) brought early closure. The combined version of PrEP, trialling Truvada, is still underway as we write this (AVAC, 2013).

The contrast between the findings of the completed trials and the FEM-PrEP study, closed early, have raised a series of questions about the research subjects in Fem-PrEP. For example, were the women less dosing adherent than required by the RCT and in contrast to the participants in the other PrEP studies at the time? Soon after the results were announced, Mitchell Warren of the AIDS Vaccine Advocacy Coalition (AVAC) has stated that analyses were being carried out to explain 'whether the differences observed between iPrEx and FEM-PrEP are due to the route of exposure, pill-taking behavior, biological differences in drug activity, or some other factor' (AVAC, 2011). He also noted that there was an unusually higher rate of pregnancies in the product of the arm of the trial (AVAC, 2011). Although there are many questions to be answered about the specific conditions and dynamics of the FEM-PrEP trial compared to the others, we wish to pick up on the remark that proportionally more women in the product arm compared to the placebo became pregnant. Rather than attribute the 'poor' finding of the FEM-PrEP trial to the individual women or some sort of structural condition (which seems hard to do), it is possible to suggest that a complex set of relations may have been at work in each trial and that reliance on the statistical measures of infections and non-infections is likely to obscure this complexity. For instance, the finding that a higher number of women became pregnant may be due to a relationship between hormonal contraception and the antiretroviral drugs (still to be investigated). Additionally, there may be an increased vulnerability to HIV infection during pregnancy thus indicating the intervention's lack of impact under particular circumstances.

These suggestions simply point to the RCT as an intricate assemblage of multiple phenomena: to review the RCT design and the RCT effects requires at once rigorous consideration of how heterogeneous phenomena enter into the RCT event, but also a sensitivity to the processuality of the RCT – that it is profoundly indeterminate and immanent. We shall return to several of these examples several times in what is to follow as we elaborate on the ways in which the enactment of RCTs entails both a closing down and an opening up of meanings and possibilities.

More ethical controversy

We now turn to the early controversy about PrEP trials in order to suggest that closer attention to the opposition to the trials might have averted costly expenditure, and at least some of the new infections, in subsequent trials. Although this seems a rather big, indeed overstated, claim, it is based on the somewhat more modest view that to address the multiple, complexly intertwined phenomena comprising trials can make a significant difference in responding to HIV. In part this reflects our suspicion that the standard ethical assessment of trials contribute to this neglect of complexity and multiplicity.

The public expression of the controversy surrounding the first planned PrEP RCTs began in 2001 with public demonstrations, including one in mid-2004 at the International AIDS conference in Bangkok. By December 2004 the concerns of activist groups linked to members of the populations targeted by the independent RCTs had spilled over onto the internet, and some members of the field – trialists, trial advocates, activists and ethicists – had published statements and comment pieces. Later, a small number of refereed journal articles also appeared.

Amongst the web-based documents was a statement signed by six Thai-based activist groups in anticipation of the scheduled PrEP trial in Bangkok seeking to enrol injecting drug users (IDUs), though without providing clean needles and syringes. The statement made reference to paragraph 29 of the Declaration of Helsinki. The declaration, initially adopted in 1964, followed the Nuremberg trials on the Nazi use of human subjects for experimentation during the Second World War. It underpins the World Medical Association's stance on ethics in relation to medical research and, serves 'to provide guidance to physicians and other participants in medical research involving human subjects'. Paragraph 29 of the Declaration declares that a placebo-controlled trial should only be used in the absence of existing prophylactic measures (in this instance, clean needles and syringes), and diagnostic and therapeutic methods. This point was followed by an account of the political situation in Thailand where access to HIV antiretroviral therapies (ARV) for HIV positive IDUs may be conditional on quitting injecting drug use. Other concerns expressed in the statement included the lack of guaranteed access to PrEP after one year, post the trial, if the technology is found to be effective and, also, a general lack of consultation with trial-affected community groups (Thai AIDS Treatment Action Group et al., 2004; Jintarkanon et al., 2005).

In response to the above objections, the Bangkok trial organizers – led by the Centers for Disease Control and Prevention (CDC) – defended the trial design saying that it accorded with Thai government prohibition on the free distribution of needles and noted that bleach was provided for sterilizing needles so that they could be re-used. They also pointed out that clean needles and syringes can be purchased legally from local pharmacies (cited in Mills et al., 2005a:1404–5). By agreeing to Thai government policy and not providing proven prophylaxes for trail participants, the trail organizers were liable to accusations that they were colluding with the Thai government. Indeed, advocates for those involved in the trial and for other IDUs pointed out that the US researchers were consenting to unfair and discriminatory policies that, arguably, contravene human rights. Although results from this trial were expected in 2009, in the absence of significant statistical outcomes it continues and still without provision of clean needles and syringes.

In 2005, two other RCTs subject to contestation were closed in Cameroon and Cambodia. The Cameroon trial, already in the process of enrolling participants, was halted by the Cameroon government while an investigation took place into claims that it was unethical. Later, after the government agreed that it could be recommenced, the trial sponsor Family Health International, with funding from the Bill and Melinda Gates Foundation (BMGF), took the decision to close it down permanently, possibly due to the lengthy interruption of its activities (Mills et al., 2005a:1403). The criticisms levelled at the Cameroon trial were similar to those put forward against the Cambodian trial. In the latter, it was claimed that the women participants had not received adequate prevention counselling and that there were no guarantees that medical care would be available to those who became infected during the trial (Mills et al., 2005b). The Cambodian trial was closed permanently by the Cambodian government and although the lead researchers – including the National Center for HIV/AIDS, Ministry of Health in Cambodia, the University of California, United States and the University of New South Wales, Australia – have since stated that provision was made for counselling and medical care, local activists understood differently and successfully lobbied to that effect.

Although controversy over HIV biomedical prevention was not new, as we have shown above (see, for example, Epstein's account in our opening, or Angell's critique of the placebo arm in the Ugandan trial), the eventual closure of the PrEP trials in Cambodia and Cameroon elicited a new initiative from major trial sponsors and international normative agencies such as UNAIDS and WHO which provide policy guidelines. IAS (International AIDS Society) and UNAIDS, with funding from the BMGF, undertook separate but similar lengthy international consultations with biomedical and community stakeholders. In a summary of the outcomes of the consultation by the IAS (2005), it was made clear that the intention was always to preserve the model of the RCT as a technology for research and to sustain research on PrEP:

> The fundamental goal of the meeting was to promote successful and ethical PREP research that is relevant, respectful and acceptable to the host communities within which these trials are taking place. The IAS meeting highlighted the four key challenges that have been identified as significant obstacles to these studies, namely, providing treatment and care to trial participants, the standard of care for prevention interventions offered to participants, research literacy for potential participants and community advocates and mechanisms for community involvement. (2005:168)

The areas identified above as 'obstacles' translated the protest action into a specific set of concerns already well known to those working in 'offshore' HIV biomedical clinical research settings. The UNAIDS consultation went further along these lines and, in collaboration with AVAC, produced a report titled 'Good participatory practice: Guidelines for biomedical HIV prevention trials' (2011).

The intention of the consultation was to facilitate a productive exchange between multiple stakeholders, mainly the trialists and members of civil society serving as advocates for research subjects (UNAIDS/AVAC, 2011). There was, in short, no inquiry into the object of the trial – PrEP or biomedical prevention – and no question that this should take place in the context of high vulnerability to HIV infection.

On the basis of the many 'failed' RCTs prior to the early PrEP trials and the efforts to quell opposition to PrEP, and in light of other biomedical prevention trials by IAS, UNAIDS and BMGF (Bill and Melinda Gates Foundation), we might concur with what Marres and McGoey (2012) term the entropic nature of RCTs. As these authors explain: 'failed systems of oversight, surveillance or regulation rarely delegitimize their own effectiveness; on the contrary, failure serves to compound and solidify the authority of the individuals and institutions that presided over the failure to begin with' (in press). Indeed, what we see indicated in the above responses is that the solution – at least to a failed RCT – is another RCT. The methods of the RCT do not come into question or, if they do so, this is only in terms of whether a placebo arm is or is not justified. So, the RCT entails its own necessity, as it were – not least because of the exclusion of the very conditions that give rise, for instance, to infections or, in the case of oral PrEP, to variations in the pattern of dosing.

But further, this necessity (and legitimacy) is additionally warranted by the performative operations of bioethics. Bioethics, in this case, is presumed to follow a series of generally applicable principles that assess and appropriately justify the conduct of RCTs. Of course, as we shall later detail at length, such principles are highly practically pliable and are characterized by many tensions. For the moment, suffice it to say that by and large bioethics is accepted as the arbiter of what is just and fair in relation to RCTs. The common enactment of what are accepted as international bioethical principles – or at least bioethical guidelines – affords a certain legitimacy to the RCT. However, this bioethical role folds into a set of practices that, as we have seen above, constrain or limit what constitutes (or eventuates) a trial: bioethics serves to exclude consideration of what the trial does or does not do to the participants beyond the trial frame. Critically, that which is excluded is precisely the specific local elements that affect whether infections occur or do not.

Relatedly, Denielle Elliot (2011), drawing on ethnographic fieldwork in southern Africa, makes the following observation:

Place, in global medical research, is at once highlighted and erased. By definition – global – place defines transnational medical research but, also in the way in which global health departments adorn their halls with photos of African children, in rural African settings (same to be said for anthropology). Erased, because in their claims of 'global,' scientists must erase place from their scientific facts.

Drawing on the contributions of John Law and Annemarie Mol (see below), Elliot states that the universality of scientific facts depends 'on never asking where-questions at all' (2011). Moreover, when those affected by RCTs attempt to ask such questions, they are positioned as disruptive of good science. Through the ways in which bioethics is enacted, it typically emerges as the prime – authenticated – means by which to question RCTs. Hence, other sorts of objections (for example, by activists) are routinely translated into expressions of concern about what sort of provision is made by trialists for those involved in the RCT (while bracketing such ethical issues as implied by the fact that an RCT's viability rests on an insufficient health and medical infrastructure).

In Cambodia and Cameroon, we can see that the objections arose from the inclusion of female sex workers whose occupation involves immense risk, including risk and/or effects of living with HIV. In Bangkok, Thailand, the disregard of the international bioethical principle that a new treatment or technique should only be tested against the best current prophylactic (in this instance, clean needles and syringes) exploited an existing ethically untenable situation where injecting drug users and others have been murdered as a result of a government 'war on drugs'. In such cases, it is hard to resist the impression that international bioethical standards are adapted to enable a trial to take place in preference to the local safety needs of trial participants.

It is in light, then, of what took place with the early PrEP trials, that we return to the consultative processes of UNAIDS and IAS that further secured the RCT model. Instead of instituting a review of the RCT's capacity to embody and yield ethical solutions for HIV prevention, these consultations emphasized the need to enlist the support of affected communities in the existing frames of clinical science and bioethics. Here we ask: What conclusion might we draw from those consultation processes? Were stakeholders taken in by the performative work of 'the biological fix' and of bioethics? If so, how did this come about? Although both Epstein (1996) and Patton (1990) provide inspiring accounts of a much earlier time in the epidemic when RCTs could be fundamentally challenged, when reviewing the contemporary organization of the 'gold standard' of scientific research, it seems little has altered – RCTs have become further entrenched. Thus potentially valuable insights available from those living with the virus continue to be excluded under the reign of the RCT. Moreover, we find ourselves proposing that, ironically, bioethics is a key actor in making possible the continuation of this situation and the corollary pursuit of the 'biological fix'.

To reiterate, while bioethics is performed as the guardian of those subject to clinical research practice, this guardianship is somewhat constricted: bioethics is alert primarily to the dangers posed when RCTs happen to go astray in their pursuit of 'gold standard' evidence. In a circular or co-constitutive logic, ethics seems to emerge alongside the RCT and is largely confined to a limited range of issues (for example, consent from the participants, provision of follow up care, prompt cessation of the RCT if results are very poor or very good). It is a range that at once reflects the standard design, and serves in the legitimation, of the RCT. The implication is that, because the RCT is ethically secured against broader context-related phenomena, a more complex and processual understanding of HIV vulnerability is occluded. Ethics, in this schema, remains an external 'resource' to the trial, an 'add-on' to, and a moderator of, what will take place – but, always as if on the *outside* of science. Despite many years of either unpromising results or indications of specifically harmful effects, and despite the ethically problematic undertaking of 'offshore' trials, it continues to be possible for the profoundly troubling conditions of life in these offshore locales to be erased from discussion of the RCT.

Concluding remarks

> What is the problem to which they [RCTs] are the solution? (Marks cited in Epstein, 1996:197)

In this chapter, we have considered a number of ways in which the technology of the RCT has featured in the HIV field generally, and specifically in relation to efforts to develop prophylactic interventions. We have shown that to conduct RCTs in this field is to be embroiled in an array of complex relations – relations that span the specificities of offshore healthcare systems, women's reproductive systems, the signification of circumcision, aggressive political regimes and punitive anti-drug policy, activist critique and bioethical consternation.

We are in awe of the complexity faced by trialists as they toil to find viable prophylactic interventions. But we also see promise in that complexity. The tendency amongst trialists has been to systematically simplify this complexity, and here bioethics has been a key helpmate, in pursuit of a 'solution' to the HIV epidemic. In comparison, our argument – to be developed over the rest of the book – has been that we need somehow to incorporate this complexity in its specificity across different cases and settings. By drawing creatively on this complexity we can begin to re-pose the problem of HIV and, in the process, allow more interesting questions to be asked and more tenable solutions to emerge.

In the next chapter we begin to formalize this argument by making explicit the conceptual underpinnings of this book. In subsequent chapters we revisit a number of the cases discussed in this chapter (as well as others) to explore in greater empirical detail and with a more conceptual clarity how trials are at once simplified and complexified, closed down and opened up.

3
Theory and Event: Approaching the Study of PrEP

Introduction

The previous chapter laid out some of the key empirical settings out of which PrEP (and the various processes and procedures associated with its trialling) emerged, and into which it was introduced. In this chapter we begin to draw out the main literatures that inform our analysis of PrEP. As noted in Chapter 1, we do not see PrEP as an opportunity – or an opportune phenomenon – for applying the various concepts we introduce. Rather, our engagement with the empirical complexities of PrEP has fundamentally shaped our thinking on how to address matters ranging from the globalizing expectations about biomedical innovation through to the localizing ethical enactments of a virus. In particular, the multifariousness and complexity of the PrEP 'case' has obliged us to rethink our version of the event. In part, all this is because in such an engagement – or in the event of such an engagement – what emerges are not simply 'new data', but also 'new researchers'. In making this point, we are also concerned with various methodological – indeed ontological – issues that arise in engagements with the empirical field.

It will not have escaped the readers' notice that we are already casually introducing terms which are conceptually heavily loaded. Terms such as innovation, ethical, globalizing, localizing, expectations point to crucial traditions in science and technology studies and sociology that address key aspects of PrEP and its clinical trialling. For instance, the innovation literature can tell us something about the technical and institutional means by which PrEP is rendered a viable intervention (or not); the related expectations literature can tell us something about how this viability is attached to particular versions of the future; and the ethics literature can tell us something about how such viability partly rests on the meeting of certain ethical criteria. These are literatures which, in engaging with PrEP, we feel we need to draw upon. Conversely, and in parallel, it is these very literatures which help us situate PrEP as a contested innovation of potentially global reach that also challenges some of the assumptions that inform those literatures.

On this score, there are other 'more philosophically-oriented' perspectives (for want of a better characterization) that have also contributed to our account of PrEP. The term 'event' connotes attention not only to the process by which PrEP is enacted and emerges, but also to the ways in which such emergence can entail the potential for redefining the 'problems' which PrEP is putatively believed to address, or rather which comprise PrEP. The term 'enactment' hints at different patterns of relations (that might comprise divergent assemblages) that render PrEP multiple. To be sure, this terminology reflects the sorts of theoretical interests that we, alongside and behind many others, have developed across a number of substantive areas. But PrEP, as we have encountered it, is simultaneously slippery, tortuous, fragmented, multiple, complex, emergent, monolithic, simple, and it, too, has had a part to play in the way our theorizations have evolved. In any case, we treat PrEP from a broadly process philosophical standpoint that draws on such figures as Whitehead, Stengers, Deleuze, Mol and Latour.

We also need to make clear that we do not see any hierarchy amongst the empirical, social scientific and philosophical components of this book. In the event of their coming together in this text, what interests us is how we can best account for PrEP in its complexity, diversity and potential. To paraphrase Ben Highmore (2011:xiii), what we value in such theory, as much as in empirical detail, is that it can serve to call forth, sometimes through exorbitant articulation, the events that constitute PrEP and in particular PrEP RCTs.

In this chapter, we begin by briefly outlining some of the key substantive literatures (on innovation, bioethics, 'science and society'). In each case we attend to those perspectives that place an emphasis on emergence and complexity. This is then elaborated through a discussion of a number of concepts derived from accounts that draw on process philosophical perspectives. What will emerge is a loose analytic framework which we hope will help us grapple with the 'involutions' that make up PrEP.

Framings

So, the framework we draw upon in this book is derived primarily from the field of science and technology studies (STS). This is a highly heterogeneous discipline in terms of the substantive fields, institutional and relational issues, and theoretical traditions that fall under its auspices. Obviously enough, it addresses knowledge-making in divergent sciences (ranging from high energy particle physics through to the biosciences via design) and investigates the processes of invention or innovation of diverse technologies (from exotic nanotechnologies to humble bicycles and sticking plasters). Cutting across these are a set of concerns about the relationalities associated with forms of epistemic and material emergence. Thus, within STS there is an interest in, for example, the role of relations amongst different disciplines, or between science and society, or the present and the future, or the human and the nonhuman in the making of particular knowledges or technologies. Theoretically, STS straddles numerous perspectives that include social realist, radical relativist, feminist and postcolonial (in all their variegation), speculative materialist. These are aligned, not unproblematically, with such sub-disciplinary 'traditions' (though these are not always easily distinguishable) as ethnomethodology, process philosophy, neo-marxist social theory and quantitative social science.

Our (hardly singular) path through this nexus of initiatives and interventions is a not unfamiliar one – though, to reiterate, it is one driven as much by our encounter with PrEP and its complex operations as with any 'rarified' theoretical interest. At the simplest substantive level, we are interested in the production of a particular sort of medical technology – a combination of drugs incorporated within the PrEP pill. This means we are also concerned with the means by which this pill is constituted as effective, as safe, as distributable, as controversial, as holding promise, as an object of study, as a singular thing, as the embodiment of scientific excellence. Needless to say, the closer one looks at PrEP, the more characterizations – or rather eventuations – that are encountered. Very rapidly there is a proliferation of empirical studies and topic-orientations that seem relevant. As with any study, choices have to be made and issues and approaches that are pertinent have to be left by the analytic wayside.

The empirical core of this book is thus delimited by the ways in which PrEP is in the process of emergence as a prophylactic intervention in the HIV epidemic, mainly through the medium of randomized control trials. In focusing upon RCTs, we attempt to show how these entail highly complex relationalities. These include the relationalities: between different professions and practitioners (for instance, the negotiations over how demarcations are drawn between the epistemic and the ethical aspects of trials); between patient groups and experts (for instance, how the conduct of RCTs maps onto, or in some way fails to meet, ostensibly common ethical criteria that are in practice interpretatively pliable); between 'local' and 'global' manifestations of ethical and epistemic accountings of HIV and PrEP; between the current (though rapidly developing) state of knowledge about PrEP and the futures and expectations associated with it. From these examples of PrEP's relationalities, it should be apparent that there are a number of literatures relevant to our project. Given that PrEP emerges out of a complex, agonistic process of innovation, which is tied to particular and contested visions of the future, we will need to draw on parts of the extensive literature on innovation process and the burgeoning field of sociology of expectations. Part of this contestation revolves around the role of ethics in demarcating what is 'permissible' or acceptable in that part of the innovation process in which we are interested, namely randomized control trialling. We thus consider the relevant debates on ethics as both a sociologically and politically important element in the innovation of PrEP, but also as a useful source of arguments for rethinking 'innovation'. If the innovation of 'PrEP' has been tied to a particular biomedical and ethical technology, the RCT, the process of innovation has been serially challenged by various 'local' patient groups (though we should also note that this seems to be changing in recent times). That is to say, the relationalities between experts and lay people are central to the enactment of PrEP and RCTs. We will thus need to examine those literatures that address this dynamic – a literature that has been called the 'public understanding of science and technology' or 'science and society'. This will furnish a sense of how the divides between experts and laypeople and, relatedly, the global and the standardized, and the local and the particular, are profoundly problematic.

Notice that in this brief overview of relevant themes and literatures, we have tacitly drawn attention to the array of actors that are involved in the 'innovation' of PrEP through RCTs. However, such 'innovation' is not a singular process. Different actors feature in different RCTs – not only different experts and publics, but also different bodies, different sexual practices, different political regimes and medical resources. In each instantiation or enactment, or what we shall call eventuation, of PrEP, there is a different PrEP that emerges, that partially recapitulates other PrEPs, but also diverges from them (the same applies no less to the virus of HIV, to the ethics of RCTs, and to the RCTs themselves). This 'multiple ontology' (Mol, 2002) of PrEP is key to our analysis. In theorizing the variable combinations of entities that comprise the varying eventuations of PrEP in RCTs, we draw upon a long lineage of process-oriented analysis that includes the works of Serres, Latour,

Stengers, Whitehead and Deleuze. We are also interested in the way that this type of analytic sensibility allows for a number of other issues to be foregrounded. For instance, the multiple versions of PrEP that emerge in different trials have, on occasion, to be brought together to enact a singular version of PrEP. How is this managed?

The point raised above – that the distinctions between experts and laypeople are challenged – suggests that the entities that enter into the eventuation of PrEP might themselves change – become-with one another – in the process. What are the shifting 'identities' amongst experts and laypeople, bodies and practices, and what are the implications of these dynamics for thinking about the conduct of RCTs? Relatedly, the eventuation of PrEP is not a sort of snapshot: it draws from a past and opens out onto a future – what are the 'virtualities' or prospects that might unfold in such eventuations? Finally, in keeping with this notion of eventuation, we need to attend to the ways in which our own engagements with, and accountings of, PrEP and RCTs are themselves particular eventuations that embody the sort of issues we have touched upon immediately above.

In what follows, we situate ourselves in relation to three blocs of literature that are particularly relevant for our analysis of PrEP. The literatures on innovation and expectation tell us something about the complexity by which the innovation that PrEP might be 'accomplished' (or not). Secondly, to engage with the debates over the role and status of bioethics is to trace an increasingly central component in biomedical innovation – a component that is fundamentally concerned with who can have voice in determining the ethics of this or that biomedical innovation or intervention (in the present case, this is the PrEP RCT). 'Who can have voice' is also core to the third field, namely 'science and society' with its focus upon the ways in which non-experts might impact upon the knowledge-making processes of technoscience (for instance, the interjections of patient groups regarding the validity of trial results). Together, these three blocs of literature draw our attention to different but related aspects of the event of PrEP RCTs. Finally, we turn to our pivotal notions of 'event' and 'eventuation', locating these within the more process-oriented traditions of STS. The chapter ends with a review of our corpus of data and the methods used in deriving it.

Innovation and Expectation

In some ways PrEP can be regarded as a minor potential innovation insofar as it does not apparently entail the invention of a new pharmaceutical compound or of an ostensibly transformative biomedical technology. As a repurposing of pre-existing drugs that are taken at different temporal points (pre-exposure to 'the' virus), it could be likened 'merely' to a new regimen that carries little of the fascination that is commonly associated with more 'exotic' potential interventions (for example, stem cell-related therapies). Of course, this is a very peculiar and contingent fascination born of a biomedical and bioscientific framing that values particular forms of technoscientific novelty and promise (as well as economic and political futures – see Gottweis et al., 2009; Salter and Faulkner, 2011). However, for all of PrEP's seemingly relative ordinariness (in some senses it can be likened to the once-a-day-ness of the contraceptive pill), it nevertheless does mediate a series of novelties. This is not surprising given that many mundane objects can be generative of novelty (for example, Michael, 2000), while many exotic things can be rendered ordinary (and less threatening, say) by being attached to the most unremarkable of ends (for example, standard forms of consumption).

Given that PrEP, at the time of writing, is still an entity in-the-making, that is, is in the process of being established as a bona fide innovation, we examine how its complex novelty emerges in relation to its testing in randomized control trials. On this score, we are interested in the process of its 'innovation' where innovation connotes not simply the rendering of PrEP as a new effective biomedical intervention in the HIV pandemic (in standard linear innovation mode), but rather signals the ways in which the making of PrEP also presupposes, plays off and institutes a series of other 'new' conditions and relations, not all of which are positive for those at risk of HIV (Barry, 2001).

In mentioning 'standard linear innovation' we refer to a longstanding if hotly contested and profoundly contingent model of innovation (see, for example, Godin, 2006) in which, generally speaking, innovation is seen to emerge in a progression that takes something like the following form:

Basic research → Applied research → Development → (Production and) Diffusion.

(Godin, 2006:639)

If we were to situate our discussion of PrEP within this model, we suppose it would straddle moments of applied research and development. We say 'suppose' because, it is very difficult to apply such a model, and not simply to our particular case. There are numerous critiques of, and alternatives to, this model (of many examples, see Geels, 2004; Keating and Cambrosio, 2003).

A key problem is that it is routinely and increasingly impossible to disambiguate basic and applied research. A simple example can be found in the way that funding applications for 'pure' science, not least in the biosciences, are routinely laced with promissory notes about future applications – and this for all sorts of reasons, regulatory and bioethical, as well as economic and utilitarian. This blurring is grounded in the broader demands placed on science by governments, corporations, and indeed publics (see, for example, Pickstone, 2000; Nowotny et al., 2001).

From recent theorizations of innovation, we wish to draw out a number of key themes that seem particularly helpful in thinking PrEP RCTs. Now a key insight derived from science and technology studies of innovation, is that innovation necessarily implies the production not only of a new intervention, artefact or system but also of the environment into which these enter and in which they must operate (see, for example, Brown and Webster, 2004). There is what Arie Rip (2002) would call a co-evolution between technology and society.

However, we would, along with many scholars, want to insist that this process is highly complex spatially and temporally (separated here for ease of exposition). Spatially, we might ask who, what and where are implicated in the establishment of an innovation – or, more in keeping with our processual ethos (see below), how does the innovation process entail particular forms of spatialization? Temporally, we might ask when does innovation take place – or again, in keeping with our general perspective, what sorts of temporalizations are involved in processes of innovation?

To ensure an innovation 'works', it is necessary that it inhabits an environment that can enable this 'workingness'. However, this environment is not one that is entered innocently: innovations emerge out of and enter into environments that sustain them (infrastructurally, professionally, institutionally, administratively, economically, bodily, etc.). In the making of an innovation the innovators must at once align the actors and resources that enable that innovation to be successfully produced and consumed (Bijker, 1995; Callon, 1986a). Of course, there is no guarantee of success, not least because the functions of innovations can be subverted at the point of use or consumption (which might also be a part of 'development' in the case of RCTs); that is to say, the distinctions between applied research, development and dissemination are by no means stable (Cowan, 1987; Akrich, 1992).

Another way of articulating this is in terms of trust. As Webster (2002) notes, innovations, like 'facts', are also assessed in terms of the trustworthiness of their sources. However, the sources are themselves complex spanning both the specific or local institutions and a general or global endeavour of innovation (or what Michael, 1992, has called science-in-particular and science-in-general). Thus an RCT might be associated at once positively with locally trusted practitioners and negatively with globe-spanning corporations. This raises the issue of who (and indeed what) has voice in an innovation process. Nowadays it is commonplace to advocate that users also need to enter into the innovation process (and, of course, there are many examples where this seems to be taking place, for example in relation to more or less 'upstream' public engagement with science and technology; see for example, Wynne, 2006). As Joly et al. (2010) note, innovation is increasingly seen as a distributed process, indeed one that can entail collective experimentation (see below for an additional discussion of this). The point here is that there are many sites and scales that are mobilized and, in the chapters that follow, we will have reason to consider a variety of these, not least the 'global' and 'local', and how they enfold each other topologically. In other words, we aim to show how in the attempted 'innovation' of PrEP through RCTs competing spatializations or, rather, topologizations that link varying sites and scales, are eventuated.

Now, in the foregoing we have, on occasion, veered toward the assumption that innovation is self-evident. Yet, as we have also argued above, innovation is never a unidimensional process. Not only do changes beyond the innovative technology need to be instituted in order to allow an innovation to 'work', but that 'workingness' operates on several different levels and along several different temporalities. The notion of 'side-effects' neatly captures this, especially when it is extended beyond the ostensibly medical to the social and institutional. This suggests that our analytic focus should be directed less toward the evidence of innovation in reducing risk of HIV infection and more toward the 'eventuation' of PrEP RCTs in which are embroiled claims and counterclaims about 'technical' innovation, social change, trustworthy voice, possible futures, effectiveness, ethics, and so on (Barry, 2001).

This approach would also encompass an important aspect of the literature on innovation, namely, temporality. As hinted above, 'innovations' emerge when the 'time is right', though the 'right time' is also, in part, made. Analysts of innovation have numerous terms with which to address this (platform, path-dependency, landscape, kairos, for example). Within our conceptual schema, we would simply say that what can go with what in the particular eventuation of an artefact such as PrEP is limited – there is, in other words, an element of teleology in the emergence of the new (Whitehead, 1978). We will elaborate on this below where we set out our approach more formally. Suffice it to say for the moment that our analytic reading of the processes of eventuation is ethically charged. In addressing the event of innovation, or better, 'emergence', we therefore need to reflect on what model of the 'event' we are deploying.

Further, crucial to the innovation process is that it cannot be separated from accounts of innovation: claims and counter-claims abound in the eventuation of a 'new' or innovative artefact. These discourses or enunciations draw on a range of temporal motifs and as such they address not only whether an emergent technology is indeed 'new' but also the quality of that 'newness'. Sometimes, it is important to stress the roots of an emerging technology in traditional techniques (see for example, Plein, 1991), sometimes to highlight its apparent radical novelty. Sometimes expectations that are associated with a process of innovation are seen as a source of hope; sometimes they are damned as hype (see, for example, Brown, 2003). Sometimes innovations are related to futures that display different dynamics, are highly variegated and multifactorial, presented with differing degrees of clarity or vagueness, and are more or less reflexively situated against prior futures and their patterns of fruition (see, for example, Borup et al., 2006; Brown et al., 2000; Michael, 2006; Brown and Michael, 2003). The point of all this is that we will also need to examine the contested futures that are brought to bear– that is, how they are performatively influential – in the eventuation of PrEP RCTs.

As noted above, an increasingly important component in the process of innovation and its evaluation, especially in the biosciences, is bioethics. We now turn to this.

Bioethics on the move

In trying to pin down what bioethics 'is' we were met with a frustrating panoply of framings. There are several routes toward this 'pinning down'. We could go down the definitional path. In his sophisticated analysis of the relation of bioethics to social science, Daniel Callahan (1999:276) writes that '(B)ioethics has as its main task the determination, so far as that is possible, of what is right and wrong, good and bad, about the scientific developments and technological deployments of biomedicine.' Alternatively, we might seek to characterize bioethics in terms of its component professional or practical sub-specialisms. As John Evans (2006:214) phrases it this:

split(s) bioethics debates into three categories: foundational, clinical, and public. Foundational bioethics discusses how the debates about issues such as genetic engineering are related to broader societal concerns such as systems of ethics, democratic practice, and the like.... Clinical bioethical debate concerns the ethics of interactions with patients in hospitals or in research studies.... Public bioethics is ultimately concerned with setting policies (governmental or otherwise) that will be generally applied to all people in the country.

Yet each of these broad brush and encompassing accounts becomes problematized when we situate bioethics historically. In his contribution to the 25th Anniversary edition of the journal *Bioethics*, Nathan Emmerich (2011:118) writes 'the past and present of bioethics is multiple. The various and varying historical narratives demonstrate that there is no single account of what bioethics is.'

Of course, we should not be so surprised at this contestability and multiplicity: this is chronic to any reflexive, academic enterprise. Or, to put it another way, the 'pinning down' of any discipline (even when that amounts to a declaration that there can be no pinning down) is also its enactment – the attempted making, or performance, of the discipline that hopefully will shape both its present and future.

So where does that leave us in trying to think the role of bioethics in regard to PrEP? Given that we are interested in the ways in which bioethics features in the design and implementation of the randomized clinical trialling of PrEP in 'offshore' sites, then it would seem that we are concerned with Evans' 'Clinical bioethical debate' not least as it relates to 'research studies'. To be sure, there are many complex debates about how bioethics should inform the conduct of such research studies or, in our case, RCTs. A key point of contention is that of clinical equipoise – a proposed principle for the assessment of the warrantability of RCTs. According to Freedman in his influential 1987 paper 'Equipoise and the Ethics of Clinical Research', clinical equipoise refers to a state of uncertainty within a community of clinicians or clinical researchers, where different groups disagree 'over what treatment is preferred for patients in a defined population P' (1987:143). If clinical equipoise means that 'there is no consensus within the expert clinical community about the comparative merits of the alternatives to be tested' (1987:144), then it is ethical to conduct the clinical trial if, successfully conducted, the results are 'convincing enough to resolve the dispute among clinicians' (1987:144).

However, clinical equipoise has not been without its sceptics. Indeed, it has been subjected to considerable critical scrutiny. For example, London (2007) in his wide-ranging discussion notes how the meaning of clinical equipoise has not only been contested but has proliferated in ways that have made it unwieldy. For instance, there is now a range of conceptualizations of the community that is uncertain about the merits of alternative treatments. Questions are now posed as to whether 'community' should be limited to expert clinicians, or include other relevant actors, notably patients, their relatives, and even 'society' more broadly? Interestingly, this concern is reminiscent of Harry Collins' (1985) analysis of the core set (the group of scientists who take up antagonistic positions in relation to scientific controversy) and the processes by which such scientists (and others) are included or excluded from that core set. According to Collins, the controversy cannot be settled through experiment because any experiment is inherently controvertible. In the context of RCTs, deriving the efficacy of an intervention is always intrinsically problematic because any trial can be problematized. We see this echoed in the observation by London (2007) that it is not always clear as to what counts as the evidence that disrupts equipoise: does it pertain to a specific, highly delineated clinical endpoint or to broader outcomes or factors that might include side-effects or ease of treatment access? Further, with reference to the various examples presented in Chapter 2, we might ask whether the 'uncertainty within a community' reflects not simply epistemic differences but disagreement that derive from the politics and economics of the 'biological fix' (an issue raised in connection with the core set by Michael and Birke, 1994).

For his part, London advocates an 'integrative approach' that encompasses broader outcomes and also broader moral values (rather than those associated primarily with clinical medicine with their focus on the duties of the physician to the patient).

Now, these sorts of debate are clearly of importance in warranting and evaluating the conduct of RCTs in different settings and under different circumstances. The discussion of clinical equipoise above is, in Evans' terms, a foundational or public one. Of course, in a clinical bioethics, these, albeit contested and unsettled, principles need to be 'operationalized' in relation to concrete trials.

However, for our purposes this three-tiered model of bioethics, which we have partially adopted, should not imply hierarchy but, as we shall suggest below when we lay out some of the founding assumptions of our approach, it reflects different 'eventuations' of bioethics. Bioethics emerges out of and enters into particular sorts of events. The event of foundational bioethical discussions about clinical equipoise enacts a particular version of ethics which draw on examples from clinical bioethics, just as practitioners of clinical ethics draw on aspects of the clinical equipoise debates. In all cases, 'bioethics' is eventuated – emerges in particular events composed of a variety of actors and elements.

Common to these formulations of bioethics seems to be the assumption that bioethics stands outside – at greater or lesser remove from – the relations and processes with which it engages: it is a 'discipline' that provides resources for the evaluation of an external, real object or happening such as bioscientific innovation or intervention or, in our case, PrEP RCTs. Our basic (and unoriginal) argument is that bioethics can be rethought as a, more or less institutionalized, set of practices that contribute to the 'making' of their 'objects' of evaluation. In other words, there is a collapse of the distinction between the 'values' that bioethics derives in relation to the particular 'facts' of the design of an RCT. As the brief discussion of multiple renderings of clinical equipoise suggests, what counts as 'community' which should be in a state of equipoise, or the nature of evidence that can unsettle equipoise, or the very character of the uncertainty at stake, are themselves matters of value or, in Latour's (2006) phrase, matters of concern.

But if bioethics is an ingredient – or what we will later call a prehension – in the eventuation of PrEP RCTs, it is also itself eventuated. It emerges in relation to a set of other ingredients. By way of example, we can consider the eventuation of a somewhat different branch of bioethics concerned with issues associated with pharmacogenetics. Hedgecoe (2010) shows how, contrary to bioethicists' self-portrayal as challenging, regulating or raising novel ethical concerns about the practice and discourses within the pharmacogenetics research field, bioethics tends toward general overviews of the issues that do not stray beyond the discursive limits (with) which scientists operate. As the title of Hedgecoe's paper puts it, bioethics serves in the 'reinforcement of socio-technical expectations' attached to pharmacogenetics. Arguably, then, the eventuation of this particular bioethics is shaped by the technical and ethical expectations that scientists attach to pharmacogenetics.

Hedgecoe is careful to note that bioethics is not a singular exercise: there are bioethicists who do raise novel arguments that challenge prevailing pharmacogenetic wisdom about expectations and ethics (though as he also notes, these tend to be ignored in the predominant bioethical accounts). In our PrEP RCT case studies, we are not only concerned with 'business as usual' bioethics, but also by 'practitioners'' struggles to widen the purview of bioethics. As such, we attempt to engage with the complexity of bioethics by examining in detail biomedical professionals' careful, often self-critical, efforts to address the bioethics they should abide by in designing and implementing RCTs, not least in controversial offshore sites (see, for example, Green et al., 2008).

What interests us is how even more 'expansive' modes of doing (clinical) bioethics – and these can be *very* expansive if we follow Tomasini's (2010) advocacy of a Deleuzian rhizomic bioethics – carry residual assumptions about, for instance, the nature of local populations and patients. The role of bioethics in the eventuation of PrEP RCTs is also a particular eventuation of populations, patients, communities, 'the' virus, and so on and so forth which are open to problematization (by nonhumans as well as humans). The point is that when we come to examine the generative capacities of bioethics that enact PrEP RCTs in particular ways, we will also see how, in the process, such bioethics also ironically serve in contrary eventuations of PrEP, in the enactment of other versions of RCTs. More concretely, we pursue this complexity by focusing on the ways that bioethics are enacted by trialists, community groups and participants themselves. So, while our analysis of bioethics in the foregoing has engaged with its 'professional', abstracted articulation in order to crystallize some of its key parameters, in what follows we primarily concern ourselves with the practical (complex and multiple) enactment of bioethics.

However, lest it appear that social science has trumped ethics, we will also make clear that we too have ethical (and political) commitments. Our own enactments of bioethics are informed by ethics, though derived from a rather different tradition in which ethics is emergent rather than external (see below).

Engaging RCTs

As hinted at several points above, the evaluation of RCTs (whether as an innovation, or in terms of ethics) is bound up with 'who' can have voice. The process of trialling can thus also be illuminated by the literatures on the relation between 'science and society', or what can also be called 'public understanding of science' (PUS) and, latterly, 'public engagement with science' (PES). Obviously enough, RCTs entail an encounter between biomedical expertise and members of the public, though the precise quality of this encounter differs across different sciences and publics (for example, global northern publics and nanotechnologists suggest a very different form of encounter than that between medical researchers and lay drug trials recruits drawn from impoverished or

minority groups in the global south). As we shall see below, these differences have implications for how we proceed analytically.

If the early work on PUS tended to assume that publics were defi-
cient in scientific knowledge and required appropriate education (the
deficit model), subsequent critical PUS reformulated the 'public' less in
terms of cognitive capacity and more in terms of social identity which
included not only a sense of community and local expertise, but also a
complex relation to science and scientific institutions. In particular, the
latter's 'body language' of certainty in its own pronouncements was seen
as key to the sometime fraught interactions between scientific institutions and lay communities. This was especially the case when the folk
knowledges and situated experiences of the laypeople were dismissed
or marginalized. As various analysts have long noted, these folk knowledges were potentially hugely useful and might have served to nuance
and modulate the pronouncements of scientific institutions and embed
expert knowledge in the concrete exigencies of local conditions (see, for
example, Wynne, 1993; Irwin and Wynne, 1996, Irwin, 1995).

Partly emerging out of this shift, there have arguably been two major
developments. On the one hand, there was concerted endeavour to
'take seriously' the public's voice in matters of science and technology
(see, for example, House of Lords, 2000). Over time, this has lead to a
loose programme of PES marked by a proliferation of initiatives that
aim to construct and assess techniques that access this public voice in
relation to specific, often controversial, technoscientific innovations
(for example, genetic modification of plants, nanotechnology, stem cell
research). These techniques – what might be called 'formalized mechanisms of voicing' (Michael and Brown, 2005) – include focus groups, citizens panels, consensus conferences, citizens juries, deliberative polling.
The aim here is to attempt to canvas public views so that ultimately
they may shape technoscientific developments 'upstream', at the earlier
stages of innovation. Needless to say, these initiatives in public engagement are not without their critics. For example, they have been accused
of dampening dissensus and diluting more radical forms of citizenship
(Felt et al., 2009; Elam and Bertilsson, 2003), or of being more or less
disguised exercises in public relations (Beder, 1999; Davies, 2006), or
of enacting and disseminating particular impoverished models of the
scientific citizen (Irwin, 2001; Braun and Schultz, 2010).

On the other hand (though this is not unrelated to the foregoing),
there are those studies that have addressed how the voice of the lay
public manifests, or might manifest, itself in the process of scientific knowledge-making. Here, the emphasis is upon laypeople's role

in – whether they contribute to or contest – specific types of scientific knowledge. For instance, scholars have examined the ways in which laypeople contributed to the arguments over the existence of Repetitive Strain Injury (Arksey, 1998) or to the design of clinical trials for HIV treatments (Epstein, 1996), or to the direction of research programmes into muscular dystrophy (Callon et al., 2001; Callon and Rabeharisoa, 2008). These studies are particularly interested in the means by which laypeople come to be in a more or less significant position to influence the emergence of a scientific 'fact' or a technical 'procedure' or a research 'programme' by virtue of the sorts of discourses that they can mobilize and the types of alliances that they can marshal. What is often key to such processes is the mutability of the divide between experts and non-experts. According to Callon et al. (2001) there are forums in which identities between the various actors are sufficiently fluid – have yet to ossify or stabilize – to generate new arrangements and facilitate the possibility of new courses of action. As Will and Moreira (2010) note, there is a likelihood that these 'hybrid forums' might reflect broader changes in the relationship between science and society. For instance, and abstractedly put, the chronic uncertainty that now attaches to technoscience (and its promises and futures) increasingly draws the scrutiny of society (Nowotny et al., 2001). The point is that under contemporary conditions, lay actors seem ever more likely to gain an epistemic (as well as ethical) foothold in the processes of technoscience.

Having made this point, 'contemporary conditions' are hardly uniform: when we consider 'offshore trials', rather different circumstances might pertain. RCTs in South-East Asia amongst impoverished groups such as drug users and sex workers are unlikely to yield the sort of local hybrid forum that Callon describes (Callon is, of course, more than aware of the contingencies that enable hybrid forums to emerge – see Callon and Rabeharisoa, 2008). Conversely, hybrid forums elsewhere, for instance at the sponsoring source of the trial (for example, in the US), might well affect the issues that are raised in offshore RCTs' design and conduct.

However, there is another point to be made here: the analysis of RCTs in these settings is not innocent, that is, simply representational – it is performative (Law, 2004). Drawing on Stengers' (2000) notion of event, Will and Moreira (2010) suggest that the RCT can be conceptualized as a collective experiment that does not simply yield 'facts' but is generative of new human and nonhuman entities and the relations between them. In other words, this characterization of the RCT as a collective experiment aims to emphasize its eventfulness – that it produces new ways of thinking the experiment (its meaning, the nature of the problem it addresses, the array, pattern and mutability of the entities involved). As Will and Moreira (2010:9) also note, this is a 'normative suggestion' (though, as we have hinted, in some cases, this may be actualized, for instance, in collective experiments that feature patient associations as described by Callon and his collaborators). We, too, will be drawing on the notion of event, placing special emphasis on its processuality and openness. This allows us to argue that any (event of) analytic characterization of an RCT event is also an intervention – that is, to reiterate, performative (Law, 2004) – not least insofar as certain constituent entities are foregrounded over others. What might be the entities and relations that are missed? And how might these slow our routine thinking down and allow us to re-envision the RCT event? Instead of an opportunity for seeking a solution to specified problems, perhaps the RCT can be refashioned as an actual occasion for reframing the issues at stake, that is, for inventive problem-making. In the next section, we turn to this conceptualization of the event and the intellectual tradition to which it is attached.

On the event of research

In situating PrEP RCTs as examples of the innovation process, or carriers of biomedical expectations, or occasions for the peculiar meeting of 'science' and 'society', we have drawn on literatures within the broad field of STS. This field has come to general prominence in part because of the various challenges it has posed for the core assumptions of much social science (as well as science). For STS and, especially its offspring the Sociology of Scientific Knowledge (SSK), such dichotomies as science/non-science, truth/error, fact/value, fact/artefact, discovery/mistake are not pre-givens but must be socially accomplished (see, for example, Bloor, 1976; Barnes, 1977; Collins, 1985; Lynch, 1985). Informing many of the studies that investigated the significance of social processes in scientific practice was the principle of symmetry. This principle stated that whatever eventually came to be considered the truth or an error in any scientific controversy should be subject to the same type of analysis, the same form of social explanation. SSK, however, was not a uniform enterprise and there were extensive debates over the nature of accounting for the social processes of scientific knowledge-making – some insisting upon, others eschewing, social explanation, especially in terms of interests (see, for example, Callon and Law, 1982).

In early-mid 1980s a new arm of SSK emerged, actor-network theory (ANT), which generalized 'symmetry' to argue that the analyst should be neutral about the sorts of entities that played a role in the building of networks through which scientific facts were established. Radically, the range of entities included nonhumans such as animal bodies, electrons, technologies (see, for example, Callon and Latour, 1981; Callon, 1986a, b; Latour, 1987). While early ANT had its fair share of criticisms (for example, limited conceptions of spatial relations, of the analyst's situation, of the other, of culture, of the boundaries of a network – see for example Mol and Law, 1994; Haraway, 1997; Lee and Brown, 1994; Martin, 1998; Strathern, 1995), it nevertheless opened up the field of inquiry by asking us to take seriously the heterogeneity of entities that go into the making of a network or assemblage that comprises a laboratory, or a research programme, or an experiment out of which scientific 'facts' emerge and circulate more or less inviolate.

In light of these and other criticisms, 'post-ANT' (for example, Law and Hassard, 1999) has shifted from a more or less exclusive concern with the linear processes of stabilizing, or rendering durable, networks to an engagement with the complexity, multiplicity and processuality of assemblages – what Latour has, perhaps tongue-in-cheek, called an 'actant-rhizome ontology' (Latour, 2005:9).

For our part, we approach this set of concerns through the concept of 'event' (though, arguably, 'assemblages' will do just as well). Drawing on Mariam Fraser's (2010) discussion of the event, we can regard it as an actual occasion in which there is a coming together of heterogeneous entities that span social and material, human and nonhuman, cognitive and affective, macro and micro, the conscious and unconscious. In Whitehead's (1978) terms these are prehensions that concresce to form an actual object or an actual occasion, which in turn becomes a prehension in the conscrescence of 'subsequent' actual objects or actual occasions. This Whiteheadian heterogeneity has been a major influence on ANT, as has that of Michel Serres (for example, 1982a). Importantly, Serres (Serres and Latour, 1995) offers another dimension to thinking about this heterogeneity, that is, a topological one. In the conscrescence of an event, the prehensions that comprise it are not 'in' space and time (in the sense that space and time constitute an external framework against which they are measured). Rather, seemingly spatially and temporally distant prehensions can be topologically folded together – 'involuted' (see Ansell Pearson, 1999) – in events (space and time are thus emergent, like everything else). The upshot of this is that events are complex affairs that can entail, from within a commonsensical spatio-temporal framework, unexpected, distal prehensions.

One implication of this is that an 'entity' like the human immunodeficiency virus, or an event like a PrEP RCT, is not singular or 'essential'.

They emerge out of concrescences in which the prehensions vary. They are eventuated in different ways. Accordingly, there is no virus in the abstract to which qualities like 'resistant', or 'aggressive', or 'surmountable' are added, nor is there a PrEP RCT that is successful, or controversial, or unethical. Rather, there are several viruses-with-their-particular-qualities and there are several PrEP RCTs-with-their-particular-qualities. And when the virus or the RCT are abstracted as essences, this is a particular abstraction tied to a particular event: the virologist's virus, the medical doctor's virus, the patient group's RCT, the bioethicist's RCT. In short, when we refer to a PrEP RCT, we are referring to concrete eventuations that are in Mol's (2002) terms, ontologically multiple. They are multiply emergent out of divergent, specific relationalities that are not always consonant with one another. Indeed, how these diverse ontologies are played out is a key theme in the following empirical chapters.

This complexity is deepened when we further consider the coming together of entities (concrescence of prehensions). To assume that they remain the same in this process of making an event – that they remain in a state of being-with – is but one particular formulation. As Fraser (2010) notes in explicating Deleuze's and Stengers' rendering, the event can be thought along other lines: the entities that enter into it become-with one another. There is a mutual changing or what Karen Barad (2007) would call an intra-action. We have already glimpsed this in relation to the discussion of hybrid forums above. At base, this suggests that the composition of an event is indeterminate as the identities of its 'components' are themselves shifting by virtue of their inter-relations.

The sense of uncertainty and of openness is redoubled when we also take into account that events are made partly through the process of exclusion: in the Whiteheadian formulation of the event there is a teleological element insofar as only certain prehensions 'go' with one another. Other prehensions simply have no purchase within the particular event. In a more topological rendition, we might say that the event rests on an 'included exclusion'. For any particular RCT event to take place, all sorts of other practices (for example, inconsistent dosing) have to be excluded, yet it is this very exclusion that 'makes' the specific RCT event (otherwise it would be something different); for RCTs to be eventuated as the gold standard of clinical research, marginal, excluded groups had to be exposed to incalculable risk (see Szerszynski, 2012; Cooper, 2011; for a parallel account see Serres, 1982b, on the excluded third).

The constitutive role of exclusion can take a more speculative turn, especially when thought in relation to the figure of the idiot. According to Isabelle Stengers (2005), the idiot – which she derives from Deleuze – is

a 'conceptual character' (2005:994) whose actions make no sense in relation to the 'cosmopolitical' event (that is, political events that incorporate the human and nonhuman – given their complex heterogeneity,
the term cosmopolitics certainly applies to PrEP RCTs). Accordingly, the
idiot does not simply oppose the event as it is commonly understood
by the participants, but is incommensurable with it: the idiot's actions
make no sense. As such, the idiot 'resists the consensual way in which
the situation is presented' because it 'can neither reply nor discuss the
issue' (2005:994) at stake in the event. The idiot is thus a prompt to a
rethinking of the event, to an escape from the event's default conceptualization. Accordingly, we should draw on the idiot's 'murmuring'
(2005:995) as a means of accessing the possibility that 'there is something more important' (2005:1001) to the event. We shall return to the
figure of the idiot in the concluding chapter where we consider ways in
which to develop techniques that enable the inventive re-thinking of
the event of a PrEP RCT.

Taken together, these aspects of the event – the topological prehensions, the becoming-with of its component elements, multiple forms of
exclusion-inclusion – suggest that the event is not closed, or completed.
In characterizing the event in this way, we should, if we follow DeLanda
(2002), see it not as a sort of 'solution' in which the various components
come together neatly to form a seamless, singular event (where prehensions concresce in a satisfaction, as Whitehead would put it). Rather the
event is a 'problem' that reflects the topological ingressions of unexpected entities, the fluidity of those entities as they become-with one
another, and the exclusions that contribute to both the 'making' and the
'querying' the event. The task – at once analytic, ethical and political –
of the analyst is, therefore, not so much a matter of accurately, or even
modestly, depicting the event (which would be itself a closed analytic
event). Rather, it is a matter of enacting what Fraser (2010) calls an inventive problem-making in which the problem of the event is recast in ways
that raise new questions, that implicate new possibilities of action.

To put this another way, the event is itself a prehension – it is
'in-process' becoming a component in 'subsequent' events. On this score,
it also embodies the characteristics we have ascribed to prehensions:
their topological 'oddity', their becoming-with-ness, their dependence
on multiple exclusions. The event is thus 'open'. It opens out onto a
field of possibilities, or rather virtualities (DeLanda, 2002), though these
virtualities are constrained (after all, the event-as-prehension cannot
'go' with just anything). The 'openness' of the event echoes the point
above, namely that rather than trying to 'solve' the event by depicting

it (that is 'closing' it), we engage with its openness through inventive problem-making.

In setting out this cumulative formulation of the event, we can see that to study the event of a particular PrEP RCT is to explore the heterogeneity of its constitutive elements, to trace their becoming-with one another, to pursue those elements that are excluded, to speculatively unravel the possibilities or virtualities that are enabled, and thus to re-formulate creatively the 'problem' of the event (rather than seek its 'solution').

However, if we are to aspire to some sort of intellectual coherence, we need to acknowledge that analysis is itself an event or, rather, a series of events as examples are reworked and new themes emerge and are refined. Thus to do analysis is also to draw in and become-with the data we have collected across a variety of PrEP RCT. As will become evident, one implication is that the 'same' component data of 'a' PrEP RCT can be taken up in several different ways. For instance, the event of a PrEP RCT can become both an example of a particular sort of protest, and an instantiation of particular sorts of universal or standardized ethical principles. More abstractly, an 'abstraction' such as the view of RCTs as the gold standard methodology for testing drugs can be viewed as both a closing down of RCTs and their ironic opening up. This is not a simple matter of interpretation. We as analysts become-with these components of the event of PrEP RCTs: thus, on the basis of these multiple becomings-with PrEP RCTs, we will need to modify our view of the event. In any case, this raises the intriguing issue of how we creatively problematize our own analytic events.

It will not have gone unnoticed that we have been less than positive about a number of RCT events and the ways in which they have been accounted, not least via the terms of bioethics. STS as a broad field has long been riven by charges that certain STS perspectives are not sufficiently politically engaged. Thus the SSK or (variants of) ANT have been accused of being open to co-optation, or capture by powerful institutional actors. This has been put down to a number of reasons, for instance: some STS analytic techniques lend themselves to their own deconstruction; analytic neutrality or symmetry means that results can be effectively hijacked by the advantaged over the disadvantaged; the eschewal of macrosociological categories (such as 'race', class or gender) and macrosocial processes denies insight into the broader operations of power (see, for instance, Fuller, 2005; Richards and Ashmore, 1996; for a recent re-articulation of the politics of ANT, see Law and Singleton, in press).

For our part, our scepticism about the trials and the ethics that accompany them is tempered by an acknowledgement that these are hugely complicated affairs and that trialists struggle to deal with the complexities they face. This reflects our 'formalistic' ethical and political stance that focuses on the process by which new ethics (and indeed politics) can be enacted. Our aim is to expand who and what can have input into the meaning and conduct of a trial event. While we recognize that there are enormous interests and huge disparities in political positioning at play, we do not see these as determinative. Rather the event, as we have conceptualized it here, is meant to accommodate the possibility that participants will be open to mutual change and a creative re-definition of the issue at stake, or the matter of concern. This is, we are fully aware, not unproblematic – potential participants (for example, trialists) might well resist (and, in any case, the emergent, creative problems might not always be easy to swallow). Nevertheless, by virtue of being less divisive, less accusatory, and because participants are enacted as open, or at least struggling with openness and fixedness, there is a small prospect that they will engage with a broader array of actors, and that creative change will be eventuated. Chapter 7 provides a sketch of one possible means by which such eventuation might be designed.

The foregoing overviews of the several literatures and the overarching theoretical approach that frame the present volume will hopefully set the scene for the empirical chapters that follow. Having said that, as already indicated, we will have occasion to supplement and nuance these when we come to our specific empirical analyses. However, before we can move onto these, we need to discuss how exactly we derived our material. The final section of this chapter turns to matters of method.

Matters of method

Our programme of empirical research on PrEP began in 2007, provoked by what we had heard of the controversy over the PrEP trials in Cambodia, Cameroon and Thailand. By this time – two years after the protests and well before the results of subsequent PrEP trials – there was considerable sensitivity about what had taken place. This was so much the case that our interest in the field was regarded by some responsible for the trials with not a little suspicion. This was not totally surprising as many members of the broader HIV field held the early trials in disdain after hearing claims that the trials were unethical. In order to gain access to PrEP trial investigators, we made use of a network of colleagues and friends based in HIV/AIDS non-government organizations who provided introductions to the investigators involved in PrEP trials whether these were planned, had begun and closed down, were starting, or were in the pipeline. Additionally, it was suggested we speak with key activists who had expressed views on the PrEP trials.

In 2008 we began our interviews: a total of 26 plus two repeats and one group interview. The one-to-one interviews were open-ended discussions and, for the most part, they were with biomedical scientists. The majority were done by phone or skype (they preceded the use of camera-equipped computers and video skype). The use of phone or skype calls was due to our limited budget and the fact that most of the participants were spread across a number of cities in the US. A group interview took place in Thailand in 2008 with members of a Thai-based protest action. Some of the group interviewees were enrolled in the Bangkok IDU RCT and had been since its beginning. Limited resources meant it was not possible to speak directly with the members of the protest organizations in Cambodia and Cameroon where other key RCTs had been set up, although we were able to interview one of their spokespersons by phone. Efforts to speak with the coordinating organization for the Cambodian and Cameroon protests, Paris ACT UP, came to nothing.

We have used the accounts of our 'informants' in a variety of ways. First and foremost, we have elicited from them how PrEP is envisaged by drawing on their expectations about this emerging technology. Our main question to all informants focused on what they believed was the possibilities for, and/or challenges posed by PrEP. Drawing on the work of Mol (2002), we were able to see that our informants anticipated PrEP as both a stable entity but also as something highly contingent and hence, in our terms, ontologically multiple. In all our discussions with the biomedical informants, PrEP was articulated as a desirable pharmaceutical product for potential application across different bodies. And yet the complexity conveyed through these interviews, revealed an expectation that the 'efficacy' and thus, more crucially, the 'effectiveness' of their object would be highly contingent. Furthermore, we became aware of a bifurcation in which the scientific development of PrEP rested on RCT 'efficacy' testing that tended to exclude what PrEP might actually become in more everyday contexts of use (away from medical monitoring, prevention counselling etc.). This led us to reconsider the problem of 'ethicality' in terms of a reduced biomedical frame involved in the problematic pursuit of PrEP as, what we term, a 'quantitative object' at the expense of PrEP as more complex and emergent 'qualitative thing' (see below).

While undertaking the early phase of our empirical research, we located a small body of literature on the controversy. Mostly this consisted of comment pieces in scientific journals by biomedical scientists and PrEP advocates along with various letters lodged on websites. The materials were consistent in their enactment of a two-sided debate: those who brought the trials into question by querying the provision of adequate information and care for the trial participants versus those who claimed that the provisions made were adequate under the circumstances.

One statement, in particular, from the Cambodian protestors resonated in ways that confirmed for us the limitations of this dualistic framing of the issue. We include it here as a guide to how we came to re-problematize the sort of ethics that offshore RCTs rely upon:

> If they [the trial organisers] are so sure this drug is safe why don't they send their own sisters and daughters to test it? They have a lot more money than sex workers and have protection if the drug makes them sick. Also if it was their sisters and daughters they would be a lot more honest about the risks and side effects. (Women's Network for Unity, Cambodia 2004)

Although the statement can be readily read as a critical comment on how female sex workers come to be targeted for the drugs, we chose to view it as a statement that emerged from a specific set of conditions: a trial predicated on precisely the conditions of possibility it claimed to be seeking to redress. To rephrase, by treating the statement as an emergent object of the research field – along with other phenomena discussed later on – it pointed to the complexity in which the trial was embedded. We shall return to this very statement at a later point when we discuss its problematic status with regard to the trial and its criticisms. For present purposes, however, we can note that initially this statement served as a provocation to consider what remains outside much of the empirical material we encountered in which the 'offshore trial' is represented as a neutral, but necessary, process in achieving protection from HIV infection for populations such as Cambodian sex workers. It also remains outside the framing of two large international consultations by the International AIDS Society (2005) and UNAIDS (2006) undertaken to identify the cause of protests and ensure that steps be taken to avert further HIV prevention trial closures. At base, then, this statement 'forced' our thought in ways that began to reframe the issue away from a concern with the RCT and its aim of a 'biomedical fix', but also toward a reframing of our sense of the process of reframing.

Invariably, when approaching our interview subjects, and during the interviews themselves, we attempted to encourage reflection on the design of the trials, PrEP itself and such issues as intercurrent infection (described in the previous chapter). However, the ethically contentious nature of 'offshore' RCTs, and particularly PrEP RCTs, meant that some interviewees directly involved in designing and undertaking RCTs were wary of us: why would a social researcher come asking questions about trial process and outcome? Some attempted to evaluate our credibility by asking us about which journals we publish in. Throughout we found it difficult to penetrate presumptions about the self-evidence of biomedicine, as if it were a homogeneous practice external to the contributions of those involved (Mol, 2002). Indeed, it often seemed that we were viewed as the equivalent of investigative journalists, which suggested, not altogether surprisingly, that the field was unused to being studied for its role in shaping the epidemic.

In addition to our interviews and a small body of literature, during the period of 2008–2011, we were able to observe, and sometimes participate in, a number of international meetings and other forums where PrEP was discussed. With the growing recognition that PrEP might be the first clinically demonstrated 'efficacious' biomedical prevention technology for use against sexual transmission of HIV, the international and some national HIV prevention actors were galvanized into addressing questions about whether and how to implement it.

In some respects the period of our research has enabled us to monitor the development of PrEP from a controversial proposition to a controversially realized 'product' ready for implementation. We have also been able to observe how the growing acceptability of PrEP came to be linked to the need to engage with its complexity: ironically, this gained us entry to some of the forums where it was discussed, and where decisions on its implementation were crafted. Certainly, by the close of 2011 we were able to witness a further, and apparently peculiar, shift in the role of its supporters who sought to move from such questions as 'should PrEP be implemented?' to such questions as 'how can communities be convinced to embrace PrEP?'

Our increasing proximity to the practitioner and scientific debates on PrEP enabled us to reshape our engagement with the field, from our initial reliance on interviews with biomedical scientists to regular encounters with a broader range of stakeholders now confronting the question of the management of PrEP's implementation. As such we are witness to a field that is beginning to re-articulate itself in relation to the process of innovation. Specifically, where PrEP was routinely posed as an innovation of global reach that can impact on the epidemic at large, it is coming to be seen as a highly contingent innovation subject to the exigencies of the local. The upshot is that we, as social scientists, potentially have a foothold in examining how PrEP can be tested and implemented. That is to say, along with practitioners, there is a possibility of exploring ways in which PrEP is not simply a solution to HIV risk, but is a means to enabling people to creatively redefine what the problem is.

In other words, the field seems to have moved on – or be in the process of moving on – in dramatic ways, and we have found ourselves in a small way embroiled within this movement, partly as contributors to the debates within the field, and partly as commentators upon it. This has meant that this book has not been easy to write as the parallel and serial eventuation of PrEP has verged on the chaotic. We will reflect at length on this in the final chapter.

The downside is that all the more or less dramatic changes currently taking place in the field might imply that the controversy surrounding the early PrEP trials and the questions they raised may now be regarded as outdated. The early history of PrEP trials might thus seem to be superseded both by more recent PrEP trials and their results, and by the possibilities of intervention that seem to be emerging. However, we would contend that there remains much to draw from PrEP's 'early period' (not least given the continuation of the Bangkok trial). RCTs will almost certainly continue, and although we hope that the following pages will enhance understandings of their performative, multifarious and emergent nature, we suspect that many of the concerns raised by those subjects sought for recruitment into RCTs will remain. PrEP has emerged as a highly generative entity and whether or not it is adopted as a fully supported prevention technology by countries with generalized and/or concentrated epidemics, it will no doubt be a considerable actor in how the HIV field views 'innovation', global/local trajectories, ethics and, indeed, the very notion of 'prevention'.

4
The Gold Standard: The Complex Singularity of PrEP, RCT and Bioethics

Introduction

In this chapter we begin to explore the 'singularization' of the PrEP RCT. We pose the question: how are the pill, the RCTs and their bioethics each enacted as singular? As such, we mean to investigate how each is performed as a unitary object or event. Of course, we shall see that RCTs, the pill and bioethics are contested and we shall trace how they are interpreted in conflicting ways. However, 'behind' these interpretations there is a commonly accepted underlying 'essence' that appears to exist beyond 'differences of opinion'. Put differently, in order for there to exist an 'essence' – here, for example, a PrEP pill that has at its core the primary quality of a pharmaceutical preparation condensed into a pill – a further set of 'secondary' qualities are necessary to explain variation in effect. In tracing out the process of singularization by drawing on a range of empirical material including interviews with HIV trial investigators we also point to the ways that other types of entities – most notably trial participant groups – both enter into the enactment of PrEP and themselves come to be enacted in particular and, importantly, problematic 'singularized' ways. Indeed, as we show later in the chapter, the bifurcation of trial participants in the form of a (recalcitrant) subject/ (experimental) body split participates in threatening the viability of PrEP as an 'efficacious' entity.

As we noted previously, we see the PrEP RCT as an event – a concrescence (or assemblage) of divergent entities and relations. While the eventuation of the PrEP RCT is multiple in the sense that it appears at several sites and in varying forms, our interest in this chapter is in how, despite these multiple eventuations, PrEP RCTs, PrEP and indeed bioethics retain their singular identity. Here, we follow Halewood's (2011) reading of Whitehead where he notes that for Whitehead, events and objects (or occasions and entities) need to be understood in their concrete actuality – not as essences that have various secondary qualities attached to them. There are thus only particular RCTs – not an abstracted or universal RCT; that is to say, there is no generic, technical system of drug testing that is applied in the specific case of assessing the efficacy of PrEP. Similarly, there is no essential PrEP (that is to say a combination of pharmaceuticals that exists outside of its relationalities) that is then applied to different populations. (As an aside, we can note that this contrast between the abstract and the situated is echoed in the contrast between efficacy and effectiveness). To speak of the essential, abstracted RCT is, within this Whiteheadian schema, to be attentive to the particular abstraction of the RCT – the RCT is enacted as an essential, universal, abstracted entity in a particular event (that is to say, eventuated in this or that epidemiologist's office, or this or that tradition of, or approach to, clinical trial design). Likewise, an abstracted PrEP is abstracted, objectified, universalized in a particular event (formulated in a particular laboratory, tested under particular conditions in a particular experimental system). In light of this, we are interested in this chapter in tracing how the PrEP RCT is enacted as an abstraction, and in particular how this abstraction – that is, the 'sense' of singular entity – circulates across different settings yet retains its identity (or 'essence') irrespective of all the ostensibly divergent reconfigurations, assemblings, eventuations in which 'it' is embroiled, or rather out of which 'it' emerges.

Here, again, we can draw on Whitehead (1979), in particular his notion of 'eternal objects'. For Whitehead, these 'eternal objects' express the specific potentiality that is realized in an actual occasion: this bus partakes of 'redness' (the eternal object) so that it is realized as a particular red bus. This also means that the specific potential of redness is not exhausted insofar as other entities can partake of redness too, on other occasions. In the case of a specific RCT, we can say that it partakes of an 'eternal object' that can be broadly characterized as 'gold standard-ness'. So, when the eternal object 'gold standard-ness' enters into the actual eventuations of different RCTs, as Halewood and Michael (2008) note for eternal objects in general, 'gold standard-ness' will fail to be 'fully' actualized, but nevertheless serve as a specific potential or abstraction against which those RCTs are assessed. The implication is that even though the 'eternal object' contributes across events, it is always manifested in its specificity: there is no idealized domain in which eternal objects reside awaiting to be called into action – they are, as with everything else, always particular to actual occasions. In sum, what the notion of 'eternal object' affords analytically is a handle on the ways in which external criteria that are applied across events at once retain an identity (or at least can be identified as such, manifesting cogency) but, also, always appear in their specificity, that is, in their difference.

We can approach the above discussion from the direction of another literature, namely, that of sociology of expectations (Brown and Michael, 2003; Borup et al., 2006). Accordingly, innovations are routinely tied to depictions of specific futures (for instance, xenotransplantation is tied to a future in which organ transplantation is not limited by the scarcity of human donors). In the case of PrEP, it is tied to a particular positive future in which the risk of HIV infection is dramatically reduced and ultimately eradicated. However, for this future to be realized, a series of actors need to play their parts: the pharmaceuticals, medical infra-structures, those who are at risk, and so on and so forth. A key insight of the sociology of expectations is that these futures are not simply representational: they are performative. As such they are involved in the present marshalling of actors and relations in such a way that, ideally, the depicted future comes to be realized.

Now while the sociology of expectations has often focused on more or less explicit depictions of the future, we can note that such futures are organized around external or pre-set criteria of success. Thus, in relation to PrEP an external criterion of success is 'reduced risk of HIV infection'. The expectations associated with PrEP – its potentiality – are shaped by external or abstracted criteria (what we called 'eternal objects') that enter into the specific eventuation of PrEP (say, in an RCT) and serve to render PrEP a particular entity (something that does or does not reduce the risk of HIV infection). While we have no difficulty with the idea of 'reducing risk of HIV infection' – or, indeed with the actuality of reducing HIV infection! – we are concerned that such 'criterial expecta-tions' (the expectations that the future is judged against pre-set criteria, or aspirations toward 'gold standard-ness') and 'eternal objects' detract from other aspects and potentialities of – other entities and relations entailed in – the eventuation of PrEP. For instance, by way of initial illus-tration we can point to those relations implied by an alternative future associated with PrEP where, for instance, PrEP generates increased drug resistance in 'the' virus thus leading to increased rates of HIV infection (see discussion in Chapter 1). In effect, as we will see, these other rela-tions also form a crucial, if always contingent, part of what PrEP does, that is, how it affects transmission, the epidemic more broadly and the specific everyday lives of people vulnerable to HIV that are a key motiva-tion in the pursuit of PrEP RCTs.

In what follows, drawing on our interviews with HIV trialists and a selection of articles and reports from the HIV field, we examine this relation between abstraction and concrete eventuation in relation to the PrEP pill, its randomized controlled trialling, and its associated bioethics. In order both to avoid the suggestion of 'essentiality' connoted by the term 'eternal object', and to signal the external criteria by which they are assessed, we consider PrEP, RCTs and bioethics as 'quantitative objects'. By this we mean that in the events of their enactment they are rendered 'essential' by the use of external criteria. That is to say, eternal objects enter into the eventuation of something like a PrEP RCT in the form of criterial expectations that imply that PrEP RCT can only properly be assessed along particular pre-set criteria or scales of efficacy or ethicality. These criteria are external to the PrEP RCT in the sense that they do not emerge in the particular enactment of the RCT in a particular setting (with this or that patient group, under these or those policy regimes or medical infrastructures). Tacit here is the contrast between external abstracted criteria by which an entity, or set of relations, is assessed, and internal emergent characterizations that co-emerge with those entities or relations. The contrast will animate much of what is to follow but takes centre-stage in Chapter 6 when we elaborate it through a topological framing.

Part of our argument is that for pre-set criteria to be predominant in the eventuation of the PrEP pill, the RCTs and bioethics – to render these 'quantitative objects' – it is necessary to 'divest' or 'exclude' those elements in the event that do not 'fit in' with this quantification. As we shall see, in the conduct of the trials, numerous issues were raised by spokespersons for volunteer groups. These issues challenged the characterization of the trial event put forward by the organizations that were conducting it. But over and above this, it might be the case that 'supplementary' aspects of an RCT will mean that the trial is more complex and variegated than might appear when considering only the quantified depiction of the trial. For instance, apart from the actions of PrEP, there can be additional protection against HIV achieved across candidate and placebo arms by virtue of the very presence of an RCT in a setting otherwise struggling to achieve reduced rates. In this reading the conduct of trial does something 'other' than simply test PrEP – our aim is to articulate a way of incorporating this difference into the eventuation of the trial. In parallel, some scientists were much troubled by the complexity of the trials, a complexity in which external criteria seem to proliferate, new aspects to the trial unexpectedly emerge, and all these combine in unforeseen ways. While this complexity should have rendered problematic the RCT as a quantified (even quantifiable) object, generally scientists nevertheless did not question this mode of accounting for PrEP RCTs.

Another implication of this approach to RCTs is that a focus upon the 'quantitative object' is simultaneously a focus on the event as an occasion for finding solutions. With pre-set criteria in play, the problem domain is demarcated: what is the best way to realize the gold standard-ness of this RCT? As should be obvious from the foregoing, our task is to query this sort of enterprise: we address how it is that particular criteria, standards, scales have taken hold as parameters of a 'solution' to the event of PrEP RCTs and the public health issue of HIV prevention.[1] To bring into the eventuation of the PrEP RCT other entities and relations (challenges, supplements) is to reformulate what the RCT event is, it is to re-work its ontology. Part and parcel of this is to see events as sites of potential, as occasions where possibilities emerge, including renewed options as to what can count as the relevant criteria, scales or standards. Consequently, what can be considered as a question, let alone a solu-tion, becomes an issue. In the end, our purpose is to show how the even-tuation of a PrEP RCT is also an occasion for opening up what comprises a good question, and, as such, for pursuing inventive problem-making (see Chapter 3).

So, in what follows we will consider *the mutually supporting quantifi-cation of the PrEP pill, the PrEP RCTs and bioethics* by tracing a range of quantifications – ranging across, for instance, the design of RCTs, the enactment of the PrEP pill as a discrete pharmaceutical intervention, the articulation of a particular delimited version of bioethics, and the diffi-culties in the comparability of particular RCT results. In the process, we also examine what is excluded or marginalized from the particular even-tuations of RCTs as occasions for 'solution-finding'. In the next chapter these marginal elements are re-introduced in order to show how RCTs can, indeed, also be occasions for 'inventive problem-making'.

Quantifying the object of PrEP

As we have outlined in Chapter 2, biomedically the prospective 'one pill a day' PrEP is composed of the antiretroviral drug Tenofovir or Tenofovir combined with another antiretroviral, Emtricitabine, and called Truvada. Gilead Sciences manufactures both drugs and they have been selected for prophylactic purposes because they meet a number of criteria. Firstly, they display favourable drug resistance profiles and relatively few side effects are anticipated when compared to other HIV antiretroviral drugs (ARVs).[2] In terms of their prophylactic properties, prior to the RCT testing of PrEP, ARVs had already gained acceptance as highly effective in preventing mother-to-child infection. ARVs were also thought likely to provide post-exposure protection if used within a limited window period after exposure from a needle or through sexual intercourse,[3] and further there had been some success with PrEP in a small number of animal studies (AVAC, 2005).

It is clear that PrEP comprises many entities: obviously enough it contains pharmaceuticals but these pharmaceuticals are relational and emergent. They are, following amongst others, Barry (2005), informed materials. For instance, the 'absorbability' of PrEP depends on the techniques which can access and assess this. A relevant example in the context of this discussion is the use of PrEP against vaginal exposure, which is based on tests that show the extent to which it penetrates the vaginal mucosa; yet with regard to anal exposure, the tests on anal surface are much more difficult to conduct.[4] Yet whether PrEP reaches the vaginal mucosa may prove – as we note below – more difficult in some contexts than its penetration of cells in the rectum for protection against anal exposure. Thus PrEP's properties reflect an 'informedness' that draws on current relations – what are more commonly distinguished as behavioural, pharmacological, metabolic, physiological – between techniques and corporeal surfaces. However, we also want to argue that this informedness also reflects prospective relations too. In other words, PrEP is also composed of hopes and expectations (Rosengarten and Michael, 2009a). Some of these expectations are tested – and particular potential futures of PrEP measured – through RCTs. That is to say, RCTs are the medium through which PrEP is to be realized as a viable intervention. RCTs are seen as the gold-standard method for assessing the efficacy of interventions such as PrEP (Byar et al., 1990:1345; Padian et al., 2010).

Throughout the HIV literature there is routine mention of the gold standard status of RCTs. As a metaphor, this idea of the 'gold standard' is rarely examined. Obviously, over and above the association with 'goodness', in this context, gold arguably implies incorruptibility in the sense that chemically it is a highly unreactive metal and as such can be found in its 'pure' form (as nuggets, for instance, though these are often alloys with silver). This, in turn, suggests something that stands outside of the contingencies and specificities of earthly chemical dynamics – it is, after all, a 'noble' metal. Having noted this, gold can be chemically combined, and is produced at various levels of purity (hence the carat grading system, though, to add further contingency, this is itself regionally variable). There are also parallels with the gold standard as a monetary system, which connote stability and consensus around the mechanism of exchange (although, to complicate matters still more, there are different versions of gold standard monetary systems). So, metaphorically at least, the gold standard-ness of the RCT carries a range of meanings: goodness, incorruptibility, purity, consensus, stability (though each of these turn out to be compromised in one way or another).

These connotations are partly echoed in the medical use of the gold standard as a marker of, under sensible circumstances, the best test that is available. The RCT is just such a test. And yet, needless to say, within the medical profession the gold standard-ness of the RCT *per se* can be disputed (as opposed to technical criticisms of whether particular RCTs meet the gold standard-ness of a generic or idealized RCT). For instance, it has been argued that the gold standard-ness of the RCT *per se* is less an absolute and more a relative (especially where compared to other seemingly less rigorous methodologies) criterion of objectivity (Kaptchuk, 2001). Further, it has been suggested that, given that the RCT *per se* is limited in its application due to logistical or practical constraints, then its link to gold standard-ness needs to be loosened (Simon, 2001). For Padian et al. (2010:621) writing specifically on the 'flat' findings (no statistical difference between the arms of a RCT) of nearly 90 per cent of the accepted gold standard of RCT HIV biomedical prevention trials (predominantly but not exclusively vaccine trials), there is an explicit need to review 'design and implementation issues that limit detection of an effect'. They see the likely culprit responsible for 'flat findings' as the lack of statistical significance that occurs when reductions in rates of HIV infection within the trial population are underestimated. Underestimation of infection rates can occur when rates in the general population decrease between the time of initial trial design (when trial rates are pegged to general population rates) and implementation (usually at least two or more years later). Time, then, becomes an important mediator in trial results despite attempts to generate generalizable results that are distinct from such a constraint. Even so, the recognition that the technology is not able fully to externalize constraints such as time and that there is need for other forms of evidence, Padian et al. (2010:632, 633) maintain the singularity of the RCT as 'gold standard'. They write:

> RCTs will undoubtedly remain our gold standard in defining the evidence base for prevention programs and policies. However, to assess the purity of this gold standard, the HIV prevention science community must not only examine evidence from RCTs with significant outcomes (including from subgroups and secondary outcomes),

but must also examine flat trials and address the design and implementation issues discussed above. In addition, we must acknowledge and explicitly define the role of other types of evidence in the development of HIV prevention recommendations.

Pure gold is a thing of great beauty and value, but lacks the strength and affordability that make alloys like steel so useful and durable. Similarly, well designed and executed RCTs are invaluable cornerstones of HIV drug testing. However, before abandoning entire classes of potentially beneficial interventions, we must forge 'alloys' of data from RCTs, observational studies, and other lines of evidence, cautiously and explicitly titrating the use of supposedly less rigorous sources, and recognize that these 'alloys' are likely to offer the best guide to decide what to include in prevention packages, what to scale up, and wherein further research is warranted.

Nevertheless, for all these critical commentaries, gold standard-ness remains a potent dimension of RCTs: it is something toward which practitioners should strive. Put another way, the gold standard appends a specific virtuality to the RCT: it is an attractor – a point toward which the RCT should be moving (see DeLanda, 2002). The gold standard is what RCTs *should* actual-ize. In other words, the 'gold standard', as a sometimes informal or tacit nexus of connotations, serves as an external criterion by which RCTs are assessed (or in our terminology, render the RCT a quantitative object). Even those critiques of the link between gold standard and the RCT *per se* seem to lament the fact that this link is problematic. Indeed, in some ways, authors such as Padian et al. (2010) are concerned with its partial repair, that is, sources of information other to the RCT are seen to be 'less rigorous', as Padian et al. (2010) themselves put it. The point is that the gold standard as an external criterion serves to frame RCTs as constantly in search of perfection and objectivity, and that where this fails to be attained then solutions or supplements need to be found. By contrast, our argument is that RCTs-in-their-specific-manifestation, or eventuation, are an occasion for inventive problem-making that rethinks the issue of HIV prevention in its specificity.

Now, in pursuit of the gold standard-ness of RCTs, we recognize that an enormous array of complex, shifting relations need to be brought under 'control' so that the key (independent) variable that remains is the PrEP intervention. The following discussions will be based on a series of examples of the challenges and issues faced by trialists, and the HIV field more generally, in implementing RCTs worthy of the status of gold standard.

The bioethics of gold

If the gold standard-ness of the RCT denotes the best test under sensible circumstances, then it becomes ethical to subject PrEP (or indeed any intervention) to RCT scrutiny. The following quote makes this clear:

> In clinical medicine, the randomized controlled trial is considered the best way of measuring the efficacy of interventions because of its ability to minimize bias and avoid false conclusions. Random assignment of individuals to different treatment groups is the best way of achieving a balance between groups for the known and unknown factors that influence outcome. This may seem to run counter to the traditional medical model of the doctor deciding which treatment is best for each patient, but it is considered ethical only when there is genuine uncertainty about which treatment to offer. By the same token, failure to tackle genuine uncertainty about treatments through randomised controlled trials can be considered unethical because it allows ineffective or harmful treatments to continue unchecked. (Stephenson and Imrie, 1998:611)

In an epidemic such as that of HIV, this view of the ethical necessity to establish evidence by way of the RCT readily extends to an ethical imperative to undertake RCTs in low and middle-income countries. In a UNAIDS/WHO report 'Ethical considerations in biomedical HIV prevention trials', published in 2007, it is taken as self-evident that such trials should involve populations with the greatest need for the intervention. However, it is also apparent that what constitutes need in these contexts is very much related to the absence or presence of a healthcare infrastructure that can support interventions that have elsewhere been shown to be effective. The need specifically to include women, pregnant women, and children and adolescents in RCT research serves 'to verify safety and efficacy' of the intervention for these groups (UNAIDS/WHO, 2007:3). However, the call to include these groups does not address the complexities raised when RCTs are considered in their specific realization. This is despite the recognition of what are deemed to be 'social factors' requiring consideration when locating a trial in a low or middle-income country:

> The research protocol should describe the social contexts of a proposed research population (country or community) that create conditions for possible exploitation or increased vulnerability among potential

trial participants, as well as the steps that will be taken to overcome these and protect rights, the dignity, the safety, and the welfare of the participants. (UNAIDS/WHO, 2007:31)

Such steps are those that will ensure the RCT is successful in recruiting and retaining participants. That is to say, concern about phenomena such as stigma, discrimination, poverty, language differences, varying literacy skills, gender differentials are not considered to be part of an effective relationship with the trial candidate/intervention. Rather, they are framed as external and to be managed so as not to jeopardize proof of efficacy while protecting the participants from the potential harm of the RCT. As Auerbach et al. (2011) explain, the goal of the RCT is to assess what is hypothesized as a cause/effect relationship by isolating 'noise', that is, the complexity of the context in which the RCT takes place. But, in their words: 'Not only can context not be controlled for, it shapes *how* the intervention works in the first place and is inseparable from the intervention' (2011:10). Context, in this discussion refers to phenomena such as laws about sex work or illicit drug use, policing, lack of women's autonomy to make decisions about reproduction, and contraception (see also GCM, 2009). Hence, we can say that although there is formal recognition of the cultural and social noise of context by RCTs, it is addressed in order to be excised, to render the generalizability of RCTs and their findings. Moreover, if we accept Auerbach et al.'s (2011) argument, it seems that the findings are inevitably 'contaminated' by noise despite the pursuit of purity conveyed in Padian et al.'s (2010) statement above.

We can gain further glimpses of some of the complexity at work within the RCT and of the specificity of context from a report authored by GCM (Global Campaign for Microbicides) (2009) on the closure of the controversial early PrEP trial in Cambodia. The report provides an insight into role of the interpersonal relations, noting that the US trial staff did not speak the local language Khmer which meant communication relied on translators and that some of the Cambodian staff (presumably including the translators), held stigmatizing attitudes toward the sex-worker trial participants (GCM, 2009:20, 21).

To state the obvious, this specificity is a multifarious one: there are many factors to be taken into account when pursuing ethicality of gold standard-ness in RCTs. We present some more examples immediately below. By way of preview, what they show is that there is a conception of the RCT as a singular technology that – if enacted correctly and not 'corrupted' or 'diluted' by 'secondary' characteristics – can produce results or 'findings' that can be compared with the results of another RCT. Much, we can say, is attached to the idea that certain procedures reproduce sufficient sameness despite the involvement of diverse persons, different numbers of these in different RCTs which are conducted by different individual workers (counsellors, clinicians, nurses, laboratory scientists etc.) across different locales.

Clearly enough the choice of experimental groups is key to the conduct of RCTs. Testing PrEP is not simply a matter of selecting at-risk populations on a case by case basis: it is also important to have an appropriate spread of at-risk groups. This is explicit in the above cited UNAIDS/WHO (2007) report where there is an emphasis on the inclusion of women, pregnant women and children and adolescents. But it is also worth noting that each RCT is expected to be justified in relation to other studies that have already taken place or are currently underway. The following is a response by one prominent trialist to a series of questions about a 'woman only' trial. As we can see, the answer might suggest an intent to map the field in such a way that no category of persons already designated as 'high' risk will go unconsidered. Yet the appropriateness of doing so may reflect political rather than research priorities:

> Why women? That's an NIH [United States National Institutes of Health] decision because there is a trial going on among men who have sex with men, there is a trial going on in serodiscordant couples, in which they do not say how many of their sample size needs to be female index partners, or male partners (so they can go for any ratio), and the same for the trial which is going on among heterosexual people, independent of gender. (Trialist R05)

Although the notion of 'gold standard' rests on the RCT being able to establish a critical objective measure of the product or intervention under study, the technology of measure may be inscribed with certain interests or what we would call values (see Fraser, 2009) that are, in actuality, not external to the RCT. Decisions on who to include are made bearing in mind what studies have gone before or are currently underway and reflecting concerns about representativeness. However, while decisions about representativeness may be a response to the need to address difference or to address rather crude assumptions about how to deal with difference, more critical questions about the 'ontology of difference' might be left aside. Here we refer to the way people may be asked to nominate their ethnic or racial identity when enrolling in a trial in order to achieve NIH requirements about addressing ethnic and racial difference (Epstein,

2004). Interestingly, rarely, if at all, do publications on trial outcomes explain the basis on which such differences were assumed and recruited for. Further, when hypothesized differences appear in trials involving groups presumed comparable in terms of ethnicity, race or region (as has happened with trials in India) – for example, showing of different rates of viral progression – this may be attributed to genetics (Rosengarten, 2009:88–93). Although we have not come across an articulation of ethnic or racial difference in PrEP RCTs, the decision of who to include in a PrEP RCT invariably relies on epidemiological categories whose differences from each other also presume a range of fixed characteristics. The usual epidemiological categories for PrEP are male, female, transgender female, men who have sex with men, gay or heterosexual male and heterosexual female in regular relationships. Yet it is not necessarily the case that such categories stand for particular routes of infection. For instance, it could be that some women have anal intercourse in addition to, or in place of, vaginal intercourse. If the latter, so, then their risk of becoming infected and also their chance of being protected by PrEP may be more appropriately compared with men who have sex with men. Men who have sex with men and are not consistently anally receptive, may not be comparable in terms of risk and PrEP protection with men who are consistently anally receptive. While we recognized that trialists, themselves, are well aware of these complex dynamics that mean epidemiological categories are not necessarily stable indicators for generalizable results, RCTs nevertheless rely on such categories.

Interestingly, the intention to cover all 'risk groups' but not necessarily specific numbers – highlighted in the above statement that 'they do not say how many of their sample size needs to be female index partners, or male index partners' – suggests a mode of taken-for-granted generalizability is already at work in the RCT design. If statistical significance can be established with a category, it seems that parity of numbers across categories does not matter. The use of statistics is therefore paramount.

According to a major report published by the National Academies Press at the impetus of BMGF and edited by Lagakos and Gable (2008), titled *Methodological Challenges in Biomedical HIV Prevention Trials* – which we shall draw on substantially in our exploration of the singularization of the PrEP RCT – there are highly sophisticated techniques for establishing the statistical power of an RCT. In Chapter 2 on design issues, a complex array of factors is set out to explain how the numbers enrolled may vary depending on the time allowed for the RCT and a preference is expressed for an 'event-driven' RCT. In the case of the latter, a specified number of HIV infections over time determines the trial's endpoint rather than in accordance within a predetermined timeframe. Needless to say, and without going into the complexities, it is not difficult to deduce that the system of designing an efficacy trial is imperfect. Indeed it is clear that a certain amount of guess work must be undertaken by those designing the trial. The calculation of what demonstrates efficacy must anticipate various contingencies, for example: attrition rates in one arm as compared to another (Lagakos and Gable, 2008:69). Let us take the example of the PrEP trial with injecting drug users in Bangkok. This trial has been extended by a number of years due to failure to achieve enough 'events' – that is, HIV infections which could be attributed to reduced numbers of exposures to HIV by injecting drug users. However, when visiting participants in the trial it has been suggested to us, anecdotally at least, that the trial has been affected by the recruitment of people who had ceased to inject and were no longer at risk of exposure.[5] That is to say, the trialists would have derived efficacy by estimating the number of volunteers who, possibly despite appearances, were not in actuality at risk of HIV infection.

In a further series of sections of the report by Lagakos and Gable (2008), we find a range of criteria important for establishing and undertaking a successful efficacy trial. Under the heading 'Site Preparedness', we learn that before a trial can go ahead, investigators must address issues of longer community benefit by a proven intervention, community support for the trial and population suitability (2008:160). In a later section entitled 'Alternative Designs', explicit reference is made to a form of complexity that could be taken to contradict the extension of the RCT across epidemiological categories. Both Auerbach et al.'s (2011) concern regarding the centrality of 'context' in RCTs, and our own earlier arguments about the problems of bifurcation into primary and secondary qualities, are managed by splitting 'efficacy' from 'effectiveness'. Differences are understood as 'external' phenomena that will affect whether an intervention already demonstrated as 'efficacious' will work in specific cases, that is, are 'effective':

> First, product adherence and risk behavior are important determinants of the effectiveness of a biomedical HIV prevention intervention, but these factors can vary substantially across populations and individuals...This variability can complicate the interpretation of prevention studies using a superiority design, because the 'average' intervention effect may not apply to different subpopulations with different risk behaviors and adherence patterns. This argues for studies that can identify improved ways of improving adherence

and/or reducing high-risk behavior, or tailor an individual's intervention to provide the maximal amount of protection against HIV infection that is available with current interventions. (Lagakos and Gable,
2008:204)

Although the bifurcation of 'efficacy' versus 'effectiveness' is enacted
with some recognition that an intervention is not a stable 'object', the
bifurcation helps safeguard efficacy as the index of stability, or essence,
or primary quality, from further interrogation. This enactment of bifurcation then uses 'secondary' qualities as grounds for additional or alternative interventions:

> ...no single preventive intervention is likely to have a substantial
> and sustained protective effect. Designs that allow investigators to
> determine optimal combinations of interventions – including both
> biomedical and behavioral components – therefore hold greater
> promise for slowing the epidemic, even though using different
> combinations in one trial can complicate the evaluation process. The
> 'optimal' intervention is also likely to vary among individuals based
> on the nature of their exposure to HIV. For example, some women
> may have difficulty negotiating certain forms of prevention, such as
> condom use. Designs that allow access to alternative forms of protec-
> tion could be more effective in reducing the risk for these individuals.
> (Lagakos and Gable, 2008:205)

In the next chapter we offer an alternative to the 'alternative design'
offered by the above report. However before we do so, it is worth
spending a little more time on some other aspects of RCTs, specifically
those that have received attention that echoes our own queries about
the contingent determination of numbers within specific epidemiological categories (see extract above from the interview with Trialist R05).

While it may seem commonplace to state that RCTs do not come from
nowhere, it is interesting that the story of a specific trial – how it came
into being along with the sample numbers required – is not regarded
as especially significant. Indeed, it would seem that the bracketing of
how a trial comes to be, serves the myth that RCTs are pure, absent of
intent and capable of achieving a quantified and generalizable estimate
of efficacy. From discussions with various members of the field, including
with representatives of the funding bodies, it has become apparent that
more recent designs of RCTs may be increasingly incorporate such
considerations of 'practicality' alongside more typical concerns about

high vulnerability of HIV (evidenced in general figures of HIV incidence and prevalence). For example, the early PrEP trial with injecting drug users in Bangkok utilized a site initially intended for an HIV vaccine trial. Although the usage of an existing facility is practically valuable in terms of state-of-the-art equipment and laboratories as well as staff with relevant training and skills, this availability seems to have overshadowed the more complex political and ethical considerations. Such considerations could have encompassed the problems of enrolling people in a PrEP trial when the provision of clean needles and syringes would have been a far safer option, and certainly an option more relevant to the immediate needs of the injecting drug community (see below for a further discussion of the ethical and political dimensions of this particular trial).

A different, but related, point on the issue of RCT specificity, and the way in which efforts are made to separate 'secondary' characteristics from the 'core' conduct and outcome of a trial, is in the generating of a calculable statistical efficacy. The following quote shows how techniques to quantify efficacy are developed in relation to the recruitment of suitable participants and the particular analysis of results. With regard to recruitment, there is a need to better detect the timing of infection (whether it existed undetectably prior to entry into the trial and the taking of PrEP) in order to 'purify' the results by later extracting numbers found to have been infected prior to entry. In the quote that follows we see how the pursuit of cause/effect involving isolated variables is achieved through the exclusion of other 'data'. For instance, data could be gathered on what brings people unknowingly already infected to a prevention trial. That is to say, it seems, from what follows, that the goal of biomedical efficacy in relation to PrEP (and other biomedical prevention trials) leaves aside potentially more interesting questions about negotiating HIV with or without biomedical intervention:

> ...we tested individuals a month before they were enrolled, and then we tested them again at enrolment, and they had to have, you know, two negative tests in order to be enrolled. Now, did that mean that they could have gotten infected during that interval and were really...acutely infected in that first month before the antibiotic test turned positive? That was a possibility. With the new trials now, they're saving the enrolment specimens of all people, so in case they do become infected within the first two months, that those individuals can...you can go back to their stored blood and determine whether they had undetectable antibodies but were actually infected. (R03)

However, when reviewing the findings of different PrEP trials and estimates of efficacy other specific – that is, RCT specific – decisions may also be made on how to calculate for infections that emerge in the data but may have occurred prior to the trial. In the iPrEX trial, a decision was taken by the Principal Investigator to include in the number of infections some of the seroconverters who were found to have been infected prior to the trial (and were in practice excluded at enrolment). This had the effect of slightly reducing the statistical percentage of efficacy but prevented doubts about efficacy being raised later in relation to the potential ambiguity of when some trial volunteers seroconverted.

As a final example of how RCT results are generated through the many procedures that make up what is enacted as a singular device for quantification, we can note that even where comparability of experimental and control arms is assured, lack of comparability may still arise over the course of the trial. Thus, in a paper on the discontinuation of RCTs because of the apparent waning of efficacy in the vaccine or prevention arm, the authors suggest a novel reason for this waning. Over and above the investigators' own routine explanations (for instance, participants might fail to adhere to the drug-taking or application regimes – an issue that needs to be dealt with in order to produce robust results), O'Hagen et al. (2012) suggest there is also the possibility of 'frailty' – where the placebo and product come to differ in their relations with the trial subjects over time. This may compromise the quality of RCT evidence and, hence, give rise to misleading 'flat' results. They explain what might be characterized as a dual processual dynamic:

> The highest risk individuals in such a [prevention] trial are expected to become infected earlier, leaving a pool of lower risk individuals at later time points. If the intervention being tested is effective, the decline in the incidence of infection over time will be larger in the placebo arm because these individuals experience no direct protection from the intervention, and so those at high-risk will be quickly depleted, thereby lowering the infection rate over follow-up. However, high-risk individuals in the active arm may remain uninfected due to the protection conferred by the intervention, so the active arm's infection rate will be less affected. Consequently, the time-specific rate ratio for treatment vs. placebo will increase over time from a value of less than one initially to a value that may exceed one later. (O'Hagen et al., 2012:123)

Thus the apparent waning of efficacy may be explained in part by the heterogeneity in susceptibility to infection in relation to time. It is an explanation that has not been considered previously because randomization is assumed to prevent this effect. Yet, on reflection, it seems feasible that those in the placebo arm are made different to their counterparts in the product arm by the intervention if it is having the desired effect. In sum, the complex nature of varying risk, time, and fixed modes of calculation may produce statistical evidence that the intervention or 'treatment' is *not* efficacious when it is. The authors go on to suggest three possible solutions including the use of modelling techniques that can take into account the challenges posed by frailty.

All of the foregoing examples reflect a series of conditions that need to be addressed in order to ensure the gold standard-ness of the RCT. As such, we can see how gold standard-ness as an 'eternal object' that enters into the event of actual RCTs has to be enacted and indeed 'repaired' in its complex specificity if its status as an 'ethical' technique that yields robust clinical knowledge is to be realized. Yet, if this were not complicated enough, there are additional dimensions to the gold standard-ness of RCTs which highlight the way in which bioethics, as another singularized entity, becomes a rationale for the necessity of a trial *and* a means of legitimating its conduct.

In dealing with the specific communities who will be participating in the trials, there are certain ethical commitments to the volunteers that are expected to be fulfilled. In part these ethical commitments arise in accordance with principles of medical research set down by the Helsinki Declaration discussed earlier and, in part, by HIV policy-determining agencies such as UNAIDS in collaboration with WHO. Since the controversy over the early PrEP trials, the question of how to achieve ethical biomedical prevention RCTs has been addressed through emphasis on the idea of community engagement. In addition to recognizing the broad principles laid down by the Helsinki Declaration that seeks to protect research subjects from research risks, to ensure compensation is provided if harm does occur, and also to see to it that participants are made aware of known risks so that they can freely decide whether to participate, HIV trialists are frequently confronted by issues arising from the very conditions regarded as best suited for demonstrating product efficacy. For instance, irrespective of whether they trial participants in the experimental or control arms of the trial, it is well established that state-of-the-art prevention should be made available to participants (most usually condoms and prevention counselling where the risk is sexual transmission), sexually transmitted infections (STIs) should be treated and there should be provision of follow-up care for those participants who have become infected in the course of the trials. We include the

following quotes to illustrate how these ethical commitments are understood as an essential feature of the RCT, but especially so because of the
targeted population's vulnerability to HIV:

> I think the key issues of the PrEP trials are exactly those that are nested
> in every HIV prevention trial. Is there adequate informed consent at
> one point? Is there adequate monitoring of participants' safety? Are
> the standards of prevention state of the art being applied equally to
> all participants? Are there now – and this has brought great attention
> because it was an antiretroviral prevention study – are there formal-
> ised mechanisms to refer and follow-up and underwrite care and
> treatment for individuals in trials who become infected? All of these
> are legitimate concerns that are part of any HIV prevention trial, not
> just PrEP. (Social Researcher in HIV Biomedical RCTs, R03)
>
> ...you had to choose a population with a high rate of HIV transmis-
> sion, in other words a population where condom use and so on was
> likely to be low, and for ethical reasons you had to do everything
> you could, in that population, to drive education, health education,
> condom access, and treatment of STIs as they became apparent, so,
> you know, for ethical reasons.... (Trialist R23)

So, there seem to be two bioethical principles in operation – one geared
toward the technical conduct of an RCT that ensures its rigour and thus
its value to the at-risk population in general, and another geared toward
the local community that needs to be treated with appropriate – gold
standard-ly – 'respect'. In this apparent contrast between 'technical' and
'social' (or local community) bioethics, each are enacted as universal or
globalizing: they reflect generic features of RCTs that apply any time,
any place. However, they can also seemingly work against each other.
For instance, to offer too much protection to participant communities
would be to disqualify them as a viable trial population. With brutal
honesty, this irony is captured as a paradox: in the following interview
extract:

> That's what I call sort of the 'Prevention Trial Paradox', that on one
> hand, we are ethically bound, for all study participants, to provide
> condoms, give behavioural counselling, treat their STIs, do the types
> of things that ethically are what I call 'Standard of Prevention Care',
> for all study participants. Does that lower the risk of acquiring HIV
> when you're participating in a trial? Yes. But do some people still get
> infected in these trials? Yes. So the good news is, for study participants

their risk is lowered, the bad news for them is that some still get infected, but it's those that get infected that provide what we call the 'scientific power' to make valid inferences about whether or not a particular approach – in this case, Tenofovir – is able to significantly, statistically significantly, lower infections. (Social Researcher in HIV Biomedical RCTs, R03)

However, an extract from a publication by one of the leading HIV practitioners of biomedical prevention trials (though excluding PrEP trials) offers a rather different view on the prevention paradox. In contrast to what is suggested above as ultimately a better outcome as a result of RCTs, we find a concern that interventions that are effective for reducing HIV infection rates within the control arm of a trial may hinder a larger scale, longer-term prevention effort. By implication, according to the limited conception of ethics engaged in RCT delivery, this more extensive prevention effort becomes unethical:

> To comply with ethical guidelines, we have reduced our ability to assess new prevention methods by comparing them to the best available prevention standards of care (for example, limitless sexually transmitted infection treatment; frequent, individualized, and *expensive* [our emphasis] condom counselling). Such strategies are not representative of the standard of typical prevention services in the community and are not sustainable after completion of the trial. The complexity of the design is increased by addition of these packages to the intervention, so at best we can measure the marginal benefit of the new intervention compared with the effect of the ideal prevention package. Thus, the ability to detect any effect of interventions postulated to be moderately effective (for example, <50 percent) is reduced. Of equal concern, those individuals who live in the community outside the trial cannot benefit from high-intensity prevention services. This challenge will intensify should we include antiretroviral pre-exposure prophylaxis or circumcision in future trial prevention packages. (Padian et al., 2008:593)

Padian et al. (2008; 2010) exemplify what we later discuss as the enactment of a problematic technical, as distinct from social or community, ethicality. The concern is pinned to the number of trials that have generated 'flat results' and the remedy proposed is to address weaknesses in design that attach specifically to steps for achieving certain statistical outcomes. As the following extract shows, deriving statistical significance (that is, the technical gold standard) in a situation where there is little by way of difference between placebo and experimental arms (community gold standard), considerable effort has to be expended:

> ...and so the challenge was, you had then to develop very large studies because you had to overcome the fact that, within your study, you would be driving down transmission, even in the placebo arm. (Trialist R23)

So, even where these 'community ethical' dimensions of the RCT appear to impede the 'technical ethical' aspects of the RCT, gold standard-ness, and thus the status of a quantitative object, can nevertheless be attained. After all, RCTs can still produce robust statistical significance if the samples are sufficiently large.

Now, the pursuit of gold standard-ness is allied to what might be called 'abstracted' goals. The simple rationale behind PrEP is the need to reduce HIV infection in a globalized setting. However, because people with HIV are nowadays able to survive much longer due to the use of antiretroviral treatments that have transformed what was an almost certain terminal infection into a chronic condition, the number of infections continues to rise. As one of our respondents put it, and alluding to the genera-tive work of antiretrovirals, the need for biomedical intervention for HIV prevention is increased in a paradoxical way due to biomedical success.

> Whatever the power of the drugs at a population level, they're not currently suppressing transmission. And, in fact, it's worse than that, because not only are they not suppressing transmission, they are dramatically reducing death rate. There are essentially nearly or prac-tically no deaths from HIV in the developed world, and so every year we see between a 6 and 8 per cent increase in the number of people alive with HIV infection, and again, the numbers are the same all over the world. The numbers just go up and up and up. So we've got to provide some method for prevention of new infections that goes along with access to treatment and care. Otherwise this epidemic is going to consume us and consume our resources. So it's a problem all over the world. And hopes pinned on a vaccine have been elusive, and there is no vaccine on the horizon, so we can't put real hopes on that. (Trialist R23)

As further evidence of the complex generative nature of antiretroviral interventions, we see in the next extended quote that prevention is enacted as a strategy that can address a universal problem – the rising rate of HIV infection – yet, what counts as an ethical preventative measure is variable. If the Helsinki guidelines ethically press for the testing of a drug against the best available alternative, it might be the case that, from a certain perspective, this is also highly ethically dubious:

> The famous trial [for mother to child HIV prevention] was with AZT which was basically the first HIV drug. A large amount of it given for a long time to pregnant women because they [scientists] wanted to have a definitive result. So AZT is a pretty tough drug, it makes a lot of people feel very sick. It causes anaemia and it's hard to tolerate. Also, at the time, it was expensive and involved intra-venous administration around the time of birth...So this was not something that one was going to take as a regimen and apply it in Africa and Asia. In those days there was very little access in Africa and Asia to any retroviral drugs at that time. So people wanted to test a more practical regimen. So then there was the question, 'Well, test it against what?' Now, you could test it against the regimen that was known to work or you could test it against a placebo. So what people did was to test against a placebo, the reason being that if you test it against the US regimen, the question is going to be, 'Does this work as well as the regimen that we know we can't use?' And, of course, the answer – as everyone predicted – was going to be that an immediate, easier, cheaper, more practical course of treatment was going to work, but not as well as the US regimen. There was a lot of criticism. An editor of *New England Journal of Medicine*, Marcia Angell, wrote a scathing editorial about how unethical it was to test against placebos. And, in fact, it's not really consistent with the current Helsinki Guidelines...you should test a known treatment. On the other hand, one African said at a meeting that I attended in Europe – a European body that was discussing this – 'It's not really of any value to us to show that it's not as good as what's used in the US, because that means...once you show that, then it won't be used at all. Whereas if you show that a possibly inferior regimen, but much more practical, works against the placebo, then it will be used, and there will be benefit.' So I guess what I'm saying is that ethical considerations are relative. (Trialist R22)

The parallel that is being drawn from the example of AZT is that what appears ethical from one perspective – where an RCT tests a given prophylactic intervention against the best available intervention in order to make a choice between the two – might be unethical in a context where that best available intervention is impracticable or unavailable.

Prevention, and its ethicality, is thus not an absolute, but is practically grounded in what is likely to work in a given circumstance. Put another way, it would seem that to be technically ethical can result in a failure to be socially ethical.

However, framing this in a way that juxtaposes the technical and social or community gold standard-ness (and ethicality) misses the mark somewhat. To be technically ethical is, of course, to be socially ethical in the sense that producing robust results enable an intervention to be relevant to the largest possible population. Conversely, to be socially ethical means being attuned to what is technically viable for a particular group or community. This hybridity should come as no surprise given the very many ways in which heterogeneity has been treated in science and technology studies. Yet noteworthy, we believe, is the convergence of divergent bioethics, and numerous social, corporeal, technical and medical elements (prehensions) into this singularity that is the RCT (in all its gold standard-ness).

In the next sections, we further explore the quantitative enactment of RCTs, PrEP and bioethics while taking into account how the process divests PrEP of its relational complexities, emphasizing external, stabilized criteria by which to characterize PrEP at the cost of internal, emergent ones. As we shall see, there is a dual dynamic at work: on the one hand, the RCT serves as a way of reproducing the eternal object of gold standard-ness; on the other, the proliferating complexities of specific trials mean that the RCT is the medium for a sporadic and sometimes virulent interrogation of gold standard-ness.

Cleaning up the mess (but there is only mess)....

We begin with the ways in which in PrEP trials, the complexity and emergence of PrEP as a nexus of relations are routinely ignored or set up as a 'problem to be solved' as opposed to an occasion for 'inventing better problems'. In brief we attend to the way that aspirations toward medical and ethical gold standard-ness constitute the PrEP RCT as an event that at once incorporates the gold standard as an 'eternal object', tends toward gold standard-ness as a prospect (or an attractor), and enacts the gold standard-ness in ways that, ironically, undermine gold standard-ness. In order to trace this complex sloughing of complexity, we treat PrEP trials in terms of an idealized time-line: from setting up trials in offshore sites, through selecting participants from within a participant community, on to distributing PrEP to participants, to the collection and analysis of results. At each of these points (points which in actuality run into each other, of course), gold standard-ness (and the quantification of PrEP) is eventuated.

Our starting point is a selection of RCT sites. As we have noted, a key criterion in determining the locale for a trial is that the population at a particular site exhibits a high level of risk of HIV infection in order for the trial to have purchase. Thereafter, scientists may encounter what are considered to be a series of major obstacles in negotiating access and realizing the viability of a trial. As one researcher framed it:

> I did a lot of work with site development, trying to build partner-ships with investigators, communities, and governments, in starting new sites as we were trying to extend capacity for doing some of these efficacy trials, and what became very clear, very quickly, in the work that I did, was we basically said, 'There's a lot you can build in preparation for trials, but the three things that you can't build, that have to absolutely be there to begin with, are investigator exper-tise, community support, and government support.' And if you don't have... I mean, you can work on those, but if you don't have those fundamentally, then you don't try to build a trial there. And we went to a number of sites, we formed partnerships with a number of inves-tigators which we ultimately didn't pursue ... because if we didn't have all three of those components, then we really couldn't do the research there. And I think that the community involvement and community engagement is really critical, and if the investigators with whom we were working couldn't build that community engagement, didn't have those bridges established, didn't have a good reputation in the community, then we chose not to go with those investigators. (Trialist R04)

However, despite what may be taken to be a well-intentioned research agenda, the amenability of such elements as 'community involvement' or 'government support' is not always as transparent as is assumed, both in the above account (to some extent) and, more importantly, across various reports and guidelines (see, for example, Lagakos and Gable, 2008). The early PrEP trials discussed in Chapter 2 offer valuable insight into the complexity of mounting a trial and how the process may not proceed as anticipated. Consistent with all prevention trials, the early PrEP trials were designed to target groups of people who were epidemio-logically identified as extremely vulnerable to HIV infection. Since the closure of the Cambodian and Cameroon trials, much effort has gone into the inclusion of representatives from the target group in consultations over what went wrong. Apparent, though, from these consultations is that those seeking to mount the trials were not engaged with the same concerns as those of the targeted research participants and their nominated communities. At the time that the Cambodian trial was seeking to recruit research participants, claims were made by activists (including the WNU otherwise referred to as the Women's Network for Unity, a group comprising female sex workers targeted for the trial and thereby acting as community representatives) that the research participants were not provided with accurate information about the drug testing in their native Khymer language, that arrangements for medical care for adverse events were not set in place, and that no provision had been made to provide those who became infected during the trial with antiretroviral drugs. However, as we shall go on to discuss, the context was considerably more complex than these claims may suggest and the capacity for those affected by the trials to articulate their relationship to HIV risk was difficult.

Earlier we referred to a report carried out by the GCM (2009). This was titled 'Preventing Prevention Trial Failures: A Case Study and Lessons for Future Trials from the 2004 Tenofovir Trial in Cambodia' and was part of a concerted effort to come to grips with what went wrong in the early PrEP trials.[6] The report notes that consultations were also carried out with stakeholders in the proposed trial, that is, with the female sex workers (GCM, 2009). However, the process was fraught for reasons to do with the very purpose of the trial, rather than, more simply, with the nature and provision of information on the drugs used within the trial or with issues of aftercare. The GCM report (2009) records that sex workers involved in various meetings did not speak out against the proposed protocol because – according to an observer from a non-government organization – 'a climate of intense distrust that had developed between many of the sex workers and the NGOs in the aftermath of the anti-prostitution pledge' (2009:12). The pledge is sometimes referred to as The Global AIDS Act or The U.S. Leadership Against HIV/AIDS, Tuberculosis, and Malaria Act of 2003. According to GCM (2009:16), it required that 'no funds...may be used to provide assistance to any group or organization that does not have a policy explicitly opposing prostitution and sex trafficking.' This no doubt adds yet another layer to the complexity at work in the Cambodia context: as such, it is necessary to understand how this pledge affected sex workers. As a pledge taken against prostitution and trafficking, it allowed for the policing of sex workers and, in practice, meant the closure of many

centres providing health and welfare support including HIV prevention information to sex workers.

Alongside the work of the pledge, potential participants' comparative
lack of experience of trials further ensured the distinctive eventuation of
the Cambodian trial. Specifically, GCM (2009) noted, the status of the
drugs, and by extension the RCT, would have appeared ambiguous to
say the least amongst those unfamiliar with randomized testing. John
Kaldor, one of the trialists involved in the study is quoted as follows:

> [w]e had enough information to have a lot of confidence in the safety
> profile of tenofovir. The issue was about sharing that confidence in a
> way that is transparent and staged. It could come across as contradic-
> tory to say that a drug is likely to be safe and then ask people to be
> closely monitored for safety issues and sign consent forms about side
> effects. (GCM, 2009:56)

As it turned out, in Cambodia the trial never began and while there are
anecdotal reports that there was some dissension within the government, the government was nevertheless proactive in stopping it. Indeed,
it was the Prime Minister who ended the trial, unbeknownst to the sex
worker advocates. GCM (2009:25) notes that the sex workers had not
asked that it be ended and believed that they were in negotiations about
modifications to the trial design. Reflecting on the Prime Minister's
action, GCM (2009) conjectures that he may have acted in this way
because of international media attention on sex work in Cambodia or,
taking into account rumours that were circulating at the time, he may
have cancelled in order to undermine political adversaries who had
supported the trial.

Accusations similar to those levelled at the Cambodian trial were
directed at the Cameroon trial. However, in this latter case, 400 women
had already been enrolled onto the trial of the single drug Tenofovir.
According to a member of the sponsor, Family Health International
(FHI), the impact of PrEP had been followed up for 'maybe a third of the
number of years as we had anticipated for the trial'. While this trial was
shut down by FHI, two other sites planned by FHI were not subject to the
same public opposition. The Nigerian trial was cancelled due to what has
been reported on HIV news websites[7] and noted by Mills et al. (2005b) as
lack of site suitability. The trial in Ghana was completed in 2006.

A report by McGrory et al. (2009) produced for GCM (published before
the above cited report by GCM on the Cambodian context) also reveals a
complex set of circumstances that were instrumental in the controversy

surrounding, and in eventual closure of, the Cameroon trial. They state that the trial shared basic characteristics with other HIV biomedical prevention trials, namely, it engaged with 'charged areas of sex, sexuality, and disease [that] may involve stigmatized people and behaviours' (McGrory et al., 2009:8). In the case of Cameroon it also seems clear that there was a 'well-organised, passionate activist network' – Paris ACTUP – who participated in the trial generating opposition to the trial. But perhaps more critically, in the words of McGrory et al.:

> ...the Cameroon environment had many elements of high political risk – income disparities between researchers and participants, a legacy of distrust over drug trials in Africa, trial participants from vulnerable and stigmatized populations, and academic rivalries over who should lead HIV research in the country. (2009:8)

Reading McGrory et al.'s report for GCM alongside other relevant materials (see, for example, Mills et al., 2005a; b), it becomes apparent that the women recruited for the trial, like those in Cambodia, were especially vulnerable to HIV. Cameroon was a country without a voluntary HIV counselling and testing programme and, moreover, without the availability of antiretroviral therapy for people already infected with HIV. Such conditions make it unsurprising that those sought for recruitment in a trial testing drugs – otherwise unavailable to those dying of AIDS – would wonder at the motivation for the trial. On the other hand, it may also be unsurprising that FHI selected Cameroon as a trial site and here we touch again on how a particular location is selected for a trial. FHI had already conducted RCTs in Cameroon and had an established collaboration with Cameroon researchers who, in the words of McGrory et al. (2009:15), 'they knew could conduct registration-level trials that would pass US Food and Drug Administration audits'. McGrory et al. also note in conjunction with this claim that: 'The ethics consultation advised FHI to conduct the trial in more than one country to increase the generalisability of the data and to ensure that they would be able to recruit the number of women needed' (2009:15).

The process that took place leading up to closure of the Cameroon PrEP RCT was inevitably complicated. Initially the RCT was halted by the Cameroon government while deliberations took place over questions about its ethicality. After a period of time, the government agreed for it to restart. However, given the problems that had occurred and then very lengthy delays even after FHI had agreed to address all issues of concern, FHI chose to close it down (McGrory et al., 2009:24). The controversy and eventual closure of the Cameroon trial has been noted as somewhat surprising by members of the HIV prevention field, not least in light of the investment in time and resources for social science research as well as clinical research. The former was intended to provide insight into the needs of the participants and to ensure that the trial would be a 'state-of-the-art' prevention trial.[8]

In some respects, the Cameroon RCT exemplifies the way in which an ethics that is associated with efforts to standardize research, cannot adequately address the ethics of 'offshore' RCTs. FHI was required by its institutional review board to include in the consent form statements to the effect that antiretroviral therapy would not be provided to participants who seroconverted during the trial. According to McGrory et al. (2009:27), 'they [FHI] considered that providing antiretroviral therapy in a context where it was not generally available would represent undue inducement and therefore be unethical.' That is to say, withholding therapy from people who might at some point need it becomes ethical within a particular framing, or, we could say, in the enactment of a very particular 'problem'. Here 'inducement' is figured as a concern, along with parity. However this figuring relies on excluding other criteria, criteria more directly focused on the saving of lives. In the process, this preserves the mode of the RCT as both distinct from *and* responsive to its 'context' of use.

Questions over the ethicality of the third early controversial PrEP trial with injecting drug users in Bangkok, Thailand (IDU Bangkok) rested on the lack of clean needle and syringe provision. The provision of these, it can be argued, is an ethical necessity according to the Helsinki Declaration requirement that state-of-the-art prevention be provided with any trial. Clean injecting equipment is the safest form of HIV prevention. Indeed it can be 100 per cent effective. It is not possible to transmit the virus intravenously with clean injecting equipment if the substance injected is not already contaminated in the process of its preparation.[9] Hence, availability of clean injecting equipment would have seriously affected the viability of local groups to serve as a 'research population'. As noted above, Thai government policy at the time, along with the Bush administration's policy on the supply of clean injecting equipment, meant that the government was in full support of the trial and it continued. Although it has been scheduled for completion many times, at the time of writing in late 2012 it was still underway. As we noted above, this is due to its earlier failure in achieving enough 'events', that is, HIV infections.

At the height of the controversy over the three trials and, indeed subsequently, the scientists who were involved in the three trials defended their work in a number of ways. Those involved in the Cambodian and Cameroon trials insisted that they were planning to make provisions for adequate counselling and information on prevention. Importantly, at the time, the absence of follow-up treatment for those testing HIV positive at the recruitment stage or during the course of the trial would not have been deemed unethical by the then international standards (see WHO/ UNAIDS, 2004). So, technically at least, they were not in breach of the commonly held bioethical guidelines. As we saw, with the Bangkok trial, the trial scientists defended their trial design by explaining that they were forbidden from providing clean needles and syringes by a combination of, on the one hand, a US Congressional ruling that research funds could not be spent on the provision of clean needles and syringes and, on the other, by Thai Government Policy (IAS, 2005:17). Despite this, the trial was deemed ethically acceptable on the basis that drug users would be supplied with bleach with which they could use to sterilize their needles for re-use, and on the stated local availability of clean needles and syringes for purchase (Singh & Mills et al., 2005:1404, 1405).

In all three of these cases, the trial investigators made no reference to conditions contributing to HIV vulnerability. Notably, in Cambodia and Cameroon, in the local sex industries, sex workers have little protection from clients who refuse to wear a condom. Moreover, given the extreme poverty of the sex workers, they might be financially dependent on extra payment for not using a condom. On this account, if condoms are, under local conditions, not useable or only sporadically useable then their provision does not necessarily serve the assumed ethical function. Hence, we can raise the point that while sex workers might be an at-risk group in epidemiological terms, the precise nature of that at-riskness is not uniform across the global sex industry.

We can also say, bearing in mind the additional imposition of 'the pledge' for all three contexts, that the particular complexities faced by the volunteer groups were not appreciated by the trial investigators. To be focused on gold standard-ness and on external criteria of ethicality – that were practically translated as the provision of condoms – would be to remain insensitive to the emergent ethicality of the situation. The condoms were not simply an 'abstracted' ethical intervention, but were, by virtue of their absence (necessitated by US foreign aid policy and the 'pledge'), materially and socially absorbed into the particularities of a local economic transaction – an economic transaction that could put the sex-workers at risk. Further, while the effects of 'the pledge' against sex work may not have been evident to the trialists and, in their terms, might have remained unarticulated as a mediating feature of the conditions of the trial, it was very much a part of the day-to-day lives of those targeted for the trial. Here the 'day-to-day' amounted not only to working in an 'outlawed' industry, but also to being part of an industry where coming forward as a member could lead to police harassment, violence, and even harsher life conditions. The imposition of a 'randomized' assignment of those already identified as sex workers to different arms of the trial – placebo and candidate – may also be questioned for its ethicality. As the interview cited above suggests, testing is undertaken on the basis that the candidate intervention has worth but is not made available to all volunteers. Volunteers not assigned to the candidate arm are thus cumulatively exposed to heterogeneous risks by virtue of the very act of volunteering. Bioethics should (ideally) be sensitive to, and responsive toward, these highly specific local conditions. The eventual outcry against the trials drew on standard ethical accounts about the availability of ARVs or condoms – ironically, these are the very bioethical principles that served to exclude the complexity we have (barely) addressed here. Under such circumstances, it is no surprise that an opposition to the trials was mounted.

In the case of the IDU RCT in Bangkok, a different sort of complexity was neglected. At the time of the trial, the Thai government had been waging a so-called 'war on drugs'. A Human Rights Watch report (2004) stated that, although government policy was supposedly targeting traffickers, sections of the police (who were paid accordingly) had, by 2004, killed over 2000 people – supposed drug-traffickers – many of whom were never proven to be involved in drugs, let alone trafficking. The same report notes that this form of 'policing' nurtured a culture of terror and many people still feared that purchasing needles could lead to accusations of trafficking thus putting their life in danger. The trial investigators clearly felt they had fulfilled their external gold standard-ly ethical obligations by making bleach available to sterilize needles, which were assumed to be locally unproblematically available. Within a set of relations in which the signification of needles and syringes has shifted so that to purchase them is to open oneself up to the risk of being identified as a drug trafficker and killed, the provision of bleach clearly does not fulfil those obligations. Indeed, bleach (along with PrEP and placebo, and the trial itself) becomes another sociomaterial element in the reproduction – the eventuation – of highly specific forms of threat and danger (rather than simply a component in a clinical trial).

Notice, however, that the abstraction of a gold standard – as an eternal object – is at once a tendency (toward an attractor), an element in the making of the trial, a component eventuated within the trial, and, an ironic element in the problematization of the trial. Here, we witness the multiple ontologies that collect within the trial event as different relationalities (or prehensions) come into and out of focus. Notice also that our version of the event has shifted through our encounter with – our eventuation of – these cases.

So, in partial summary, we can draw out the following point. Once a research site and a trial community have been identified, a key task is the selection of participants to be distributed across experimental and control arms of the RCT. The testing of PrEP (as in the cases of vaccines and microbicides) requires at a basic level (upon which gold standardness and technical ethicality rests) that participants be HIV negative, so that the efficacy of PrEP can be assessed. However, this requirement in its practical implementation has implications for participants. Put baldly, the necessity for HIV antibody testing to accompany the initial prescription of PrEP (as well as forming part of the ongoing monitoring and re-prescribing of PrEP) does not 'merely' designate HIV negative status. It can also act in morally situating initial participants. Those who are rejected as participants because of HIV positive status can become subject to discrimination or avoidance, or else generate tensions within the local community from which participants are drawn. The point is that the very process by which volunteer selectivity is enacted in the practical organization of a PrEP RCT proliferates and complexifies the relationalities that comprise the trial. PrEP can thus, for instance, trigger or potentialize elements of the local that can enter into and disrupt the trial (as well as, of course, create problems within the community).

This complexifying dynamic is also witnessed in another aspect of PrEP trials. Again, this rests on the simplified (gold standard-ly) conceptualization of PrEP – the pill itself in this case. Within the HIV field in general, the predominant view is that variables – and their objects – are fixed: they are ontologically stable. This means that the PrEP pill is not regarded as co-emergent with other objects, most obviously other technologies that have a bearing on HIV prevention. For example, in the MIRA trial (Methods for Improving Reproductive Health in Africa), which asked women in the experimental arm to use a diaphragm with a condom during sexual intercourse, it was found that condom use was less likely in the experimental arm than in the control arm in which women were asked to use condoms only (Padian et al., 2007). The upshot was that the former group faced increased levels of risk of HIV infection. In relation to the RCT formulation of these preventative interventions, the combination of condom-and-diaphragm is simply a matter of co-existence, or being-with (see Chapter 3). The associated bioethics reflects this essential separateness of preventative measures. Thus, the values associated with these measures can be simply added together, or ranked. If each of these prophylactic objects (condom and diaphragm, in this instance, though it could just as readily be PrEP or a microbicide) is treated quantitatively, affording their respective level of protection, it is becomes ethical to encourage either the use of the more protective object over the lesser, or else recommend the use of their combination. Against these additive or comparative formulations of the preventive object can be set an alternative view of these as becoming-with one another, a co-emergence or intra-action. What a diaphragm or the PrEP pill 'is' – its ontology – shifts as its relations shift (and in the process we conceptually move from thinking about these technologies as quantitative object to viewing them as qualitative things – see Chapter 5). The diaphragm in its situated relation with the condom serves to transform the enactment of the condom. As Rosengarten et al. (2008) observe, combining prevention technologies changes the way they are used: the technologies and their associated modes of practice intra-act (Barad, 2007) and co-emerge – become-with one another – to produce a new, unforeseen event. Similarly, the biomedical interjection of PrEP can thus serve to reconfigure the enactment of the condom – it becomes less socially and materiality 'feasible' as a preventative measure, while PrEP in the context of the relative inconvenience of condom use (partly triggered by the novel co-presence of PrEP), becomes a replacement.

Multiple comparisons: Trails of trials

In the foregoing we have examined the manner in which scientists deploy a number of devices in the quest for enacting PrEP, RCT and bioethics as quantitative, stable and singularized. We have traced how this is linked to the abstraction, or eternal object, of gold standardness, which is complexly incorporated into the RCT event as a reality, a tendency or promise, in need of ongoing enactment, and, ironically, implicated in its own subversion. We now turn to a final example of this process – the way that the results of multiple trials are made relevant to programmes of HIV prevention. This is not a linear process however – after all, measures of efficacy cannot necessarily be extrapolated to an understanding of the effectiveness of the intervention. Both Kippax (2010) and Heise et al. (2011) identify issues that may affect the effective use of an intervention outside the trial conditions. In the case of PrEP, for instance, effectiveness will depend, to some extent, on access to the drugs or the impact of PrEP on other prophylactic objects and practices. Hence we can say that, consistent with the argument we have been making in this chapter with regard to the enactment of PrEP, RCTs and bioethics as singular, the efficacy-oriented trial – by design – externalizes phenomena that may in actuality be central to effective practice.

Indeed, we can elaborate on this: what is externalized is a partial achievement of the RCT itself, even while, at the same time, that which is externalized is inscribed in the candidate intervention that is being trialled. For instance, drugs are entities that work through a mix of nonhuman (in this instance pharmacological and metabolic actions in the terms of biomedical science) and human (consistency of dosing, negotiations over disclosure) actions. To some extent these actions are already presupposed within a PrEP RCT – for efficacy to be measurable, then a series of happenings need to have taken place. However, and this point is crucial, post-trial (if there is significant enough evidence of efficacy and PrEP is made available) there is no guarantee that these presupposed conditions will continue to pertain. As the sociology of scientific knowledge has long charted, because something 'works' under one set of conditions does not mean it will 'work' under another (see, for example, Wynne, 1989). In the present case of PrEP, this is exacerbated when those conditions are so variable across different potential user sites – where there are such differences in terms of metabolic, nutritional, cultural, environmental, genetic conditions. So although the RCT is enacted as a singular entity and is undertaken in order to compile and assess data across different settings – notably, national settings – it is able to do so only because it 'conflates' data from multiple divergent engagements in ways that effectively efface those differences.

To illustrate further what we mean by this argument, we refer to findings from a recent series of PrEP RCTs, outlined in Chapter 2, some of which included topical microbicides along with oral PrEP. Of particular concern here is not so much that PrEP RCTs have generated very different and seemingly confounding results – as we shall soon note – but, rather, how these disparate findings are managed. Despite the demonstrated efficacy of PrEP in men as evidenced by the iPrEX trial with MSM (men who have sex with men) (Grant et al., 2010) and the Partners PrEP study which involved heterosexual serodiscordant couples (where only one partner is HIV positive) and included both HIV-negative men and women (Paxton, 2012), RCT findings of PrEP in women have not been so straightforward. Although the Partners PrEP study found both the single drug Tenofovir version of PrEP and the combination drug Truvada version of PrEP to be efficacious in women at levels similar to those of men (indeed the use of the single drug Tenofovir was shown as more efficacious in women than men) (Paxton, 2012), the Fem-PrEP and VOICE RCTs have not been able to deliver such positive results. The multi-site Fem-PrEP RCT testing Truvada with women was closed down because of lack of efficacy results (Van Damme et al., 2012). VOICE (MTN, 2012) halted its single drug Tenofovir-only oral PrEP arm and a Tenofovir topical microbicide arm because of lack of efficacy results. The only remaining arm showing efficacy, at the time of writing, is testing oral Truvada. That is, VOICE is finding efficacy in a manner that partly aligns with the findings of the Partners Study in women and therefore runs counter to the Fem-PrEP trial results. But its lack of efficacy finding with the single drug Tenofovir seems contrary to the Partners Study.

To date, FHI, trial sponsor for the Fem-PrEP trial, has suggested that the failure of this particular multi-site trial may have been the result of its participants' poor dosing adherence or, alternatively, there may simply be a lack of effect of the product among women (in contrast to men who have sex with men). But the latter seems unlikely given an earlier study by Dumond et al. (2007) that found high drug exposure in the female genital tract (seemingly confirmed by the Partners PrEP study), which was presumably the justification for trialling PrEP in women in the first place.[10] FHI has also reported an 'unexpected' higher number of pregnancies in the Truvada arm compared to the placebo arm.[11] If we deduce from the pregnancy rates that women did not use contraception as anticipated (despite it being required for safety reasons) by the trial, then we may begin to see the sort of becoming discussed above in reference to the MIRA trial where the diaphragm and condom were, seemingly, co-affective in producing another unexpected and disappointing result. Fem-PrEP and the failed Tenofovir arms of VOICE reveal how a non-efficacious PrEP emerges in conditions of heterogeneity different from those at work in the other RCTs. Within all this heterogeneity, a particularly complex version of 'femaleness' emerges in relation to HIV and to hormones. For some time, there has been suggestive evidence that pregnant women are more vulnerable to HIV infection than other women and that hormonal contraceptives increase the risk of acquiring and transmitting HIV, with the highest risk amongst those using injectible contraceptives (Heffron et al., 2012; Gray et al., 2005).[12] But even if the explanations of poor adherence and/or pregnancy or contraceptive hormones are important elements of heterogeneity, the manner in which they are offered is problematic when comparing the different randomized arms in the VOICE RCT findings with the PrEP Partners Study. It remains unclear why an intervention – the single drug Tenofovir – failed when it worked in the Partners Study. If the explanation is poor adherence as hypothesized in relation to the women in the Fem-PrEP trial and, if randomization is an effective base for comparison, we can ask why is the combination drug – Truvada – showing some efficacy in VOICE.

That is to say, is it possible that the women randomized in the VOICE trial to the Tenofovir arm are somehow 'different' to those randomized to the Truvada arm? Indeed, could they be different within the current time frame (as this volume goes to press), to be shown as not different in the course of a continuing arm of VOICE? To date, we have not been able to locate any discussion on this nexus of disparate results.

The point of this account is to demonstrate the heady extent of difference across RCTs. To enact the comparability of RCTs such difference needs to be stripped down or even, as would appear to be the case so far, excluded. Across the complex sociomaterial contingencies (for example, the impact of pregnancy, of hormonal contraception, of adherence levels), analytic choices have to be made which render some criteria more prominent than others. These criteria both operate as the basis of comparison across trials and underpin the unitary or singularized measure of the interventions' 'efficacy'. As we have seen, these criteria are set 'externally', and serve in the quantification of PrEP.

As a final illustration, we consider a follow-up article that reviewed the confounding results of the trials. Authored by the prominent figure within in the HIV field, Myron Cohen, with colleague Lindsey Baden (2012:459), it argues that what is needed are more studies which should include the following:

> the likely routes of HIV transmission (vaginal vs. anal mucosa); the inclusion of established discordant couples in the Partners PrEP Study, whose sexual behaviors and susceptibility to HIV may be different from those of couples in which both partners are HIV-negative; and most important, medical adherence by study participants. (2012:459, 460)

What we find in the above extract is that, although Cohen and Baden (2012) recognize that there is heterogeneity, their proposal fails to take into account how heterogeneity is emergent and generated in the becoming together of phenomena particular to that setting. Although the relations that emerged as HIV susceptibility in the nonoxynol-9 RCT (discussed in Chapter 2) and the diaphragm trial (MIRA, discussed above), are not the same, it is worth reflecting again on how certain relations or associations generate new unanticipated phenomena.

While the process-oriented approach we are proposing in this volume is not widely shared within the HIV field, there is concern by some practitioners and commentators that the bifurcation of efficacy and effectiveness produces misleading results as it actively erases heterogeneity. According to Heise et al. (2011:11), seemingly stable measures of efficacy are products of a mix of variables that, in themselves, are not stable.

Their primary concern is how the male condom has been estimated to have a considerably higher efficacy and effectiveness than an anticipated topical vaginal microbicide. They question how certain modes of modelling assess per-sex-act infection to generate a figure of what is condom *efficacy* and not *effectiveness*, in this case condom use over time within on-going relationships. Importantly, significant numbers of women become HIV infected in such relationships (Heise et al., 2011:14). So, in parallel with the heterogeneous forms of relationality and co-emergence that we have been addressing in the foregoing, Heise et al.'s critique shows how 'modelling' – which seems to be becoming the new 'gold standard' for guiding public health policy following RCT results (even replacing RCTs as these become more difficult to operationalize) – always functions within certain parameters. One point is that even such prophylactic stalwarts as the condom, against which interventions such as PrEP are compared, need to be treated with circumspection as measures of their protective capacity may be highly contingent. The broader issue at stake is that measures such as 'per-sex-act infection', rather than rendering the use of an intervention comparable across different settings and groups, can simply end up disguising difference.

So far, we have examined the operations, promises, limitations and unintended consequences of the gold standard-ness of RCTs for the trial itself and for such component elements as the 'character' and conditions of volunteer communities, the emergent moralization of HIV infected bodies, and the shifting meanings of prophylactic interventions. As noted above, we also, however, would need to follow the implications of the gold standard-ness of RCTs beyond the trial, to the potential rollout of PrEP into other communities. The list of contingencies immediately above serves to remind us that the few examples of co-emergence and heterogeneity, discussed earlier, pale into insignificance when placed in the context of the multiple, cumulative complexities presented across sites in which PrEP is tested for effectiveness (as opposed to efficacy) or where it is made available as an actual prophylactic intervention.

In sum, the gold standard-ness of the RCT is designed to transcend just such contingency, complexity and multiplicity: it is an abstraction that in being realized through the individual trials serves to render those trial comparable such that the essence of PrEP's efficacy becomes evident. However, once we begin to trace how this abstraction – this 'eternal object' – is reworked though the complex relationalities and convoluted becoming-withs that comprise the actual occasions of the individual trials (and their consequences), we also see how this comparability is compromised in various ways. Or, to put it another way, which reflects our focus on the openness of the event, the gold standard-ly RCT (through the measuring of efficacy) is a 'solution' to the problem of variability. By contrast, we would argue that it is this very variability that occasions the rethinking of the problem, of posing it 'inventively'.

Concluding remarks

In this chapter, we have considered some of the ways in which gold standard-ness can be used to characterize PrEP RCTs: it can be regarded, we have suggested, as an external criterion – an attractor – toward which PrEP RCTs orient and move. We have also considered the way that gold standard-ness is realized in the practices of practitioners and trialists as they go about eventuating individual trials, or as they draw the comparison across trials. Along the way, we have attempted to show that this framing of RCTs in relation to gold standard-ness yields unwieldy complexity, heterogeneity and openness – unwieldy from within this framing, of course. Our argument is that this unwieldiness is an opportunity for 'creative problem making'.

To be sure, at this stage, this might seem like a rather abstract, and, very possibly, a somewhat idealistic, prospect. However, we would suggest that it is possible to detect elements of this alternative version of RCTs in various actors' – trialists' as well as activists' – accounts of the testing of PrEP. In the next chapter, we begin to examine some of the ways in which complexity, heterogeneity and openness are enacted, not in terms of a problem to be solved, but, in part at least, as a means of moving toward creative reformulations of RCTs, PrEP and the problems they are addressing.

5
PrEPs, Multiplicity and the Qualification of Knowledge and Ethics

Introduction

In the previous chapter, we were concerned to trace the way that PrEP as a pill, PrEP RCTs and bioethics were collectively and mutually singularized. By focusing on various entities, not least through an engagement with expert and practitioner accounts, we showed how these were enacted as quantitative objects: that is to say, they were stabilized in relation to a set of criteria, measurements, parameterizations or standards that seemingly stood 'outside' of the complex events that comprise the trialling of the PrEP pill.

The discussion was thus primarily concerned with how the event of a PrEP RCT was essentially 'closed down' (in the sense of being reified as opposed to being stopped). As we argued, this was mainly due to the role – the 'ingression' – of an externalized conception of the RCT as a technical and social gold standard. Here, we formulated the notion of trial event along four dimensions: the gold standard-ness of RCTs is a core element – prehension – present in the making or eventuation of the trial (that is, it is instrumental in the heterogeneous enactment of the trial); simultaneously, it served as an attractor toward which the trial is moving (as the meaning and practice of the RCT is oriented toward the prospect of gold standard-ness, so the openness of the trial event is in the process of closing down). These – the presence and the prospect of gold standard-ness – are the two dimensions that we concentrated upon in the previous chapter.

In this chapter, we begin to explore the way that the eventuation of PrEP RCTs is indeed open in the sense of being marked by becoming-with, and is thus generative of new potentialities. We therefore consider how gold standard-ness itself *emerges through* the eventuation of PrEP RCTs. That is to say, we examine how gold standard-ness in being eventuated by each trial is, also, in principle at least, open to an immanent reconfiguration: it becomes something other. The fourth dimension of the event relates to the way that gold standard-ness is also what might be called a 'provocation': it is a sort of 'anti-attractor' that orients the RCT event toward alternative prospects, precipitating 'counter-reactions' and the likely actualization of unanticipated elements of the RCT PrEP event. In the present case, this most obviously takes the form of various types of resistance to, or subversion of, the conduct of the trial but as we shall see, it can also entail a reworking of, for instance, the very idea of 'data'.

Having set out the general approach of the chapter, we should warn that, while we can analytically distinguish between these aspects of the event, in practice, these cannot always be so readily disentangled empirically.

By focusing upon this open, immanent, virtual aspect of the RCT PrEP event, we are also addressing the ways in which the pill, bioethics and the RCT are themselves fluid, multiplicitous, emergent – what we call, qualitative things.

In what follows, we expand on this at length, detailing these processes of 'qualification' in a number of analyses of PrEP RCTs and drawing again on our empirical materials. To do so, we begin by taking stock of the sheer complexity of the RCT PrEP trials. Here, our aim is to indicate how the elements that are relevant for grasping the success or otherwise of such trials (success not only in terms of assessing efficacy, but also of enabling the successful ethical and practical conduct of the trials) proliferate, seemingly endlessly. Or rather, we show how the variety of elements that emerge within and across trials challenges the very idea of 'a' PrEP pill or 'the' RCT and its gold standard status. As such, we re-consider the ways in which the RCT and its gold standard-ness emerge through the specific eventuation of trials, and across trials (where different trials are brought together to compare efficacy of PrEP across different or the same populations). We then address how the abstraction that is the gold standard-ness of RCTs 'provokes' a reaction (that is, serves as what we have called an 'anti-attractor'). It ironically enables virtual aspects of the RCT event that are otherwise marginal or 'antagonistic' to be actualized. As we shall see, and as the partial listing of the sheer complexity of the PrEP RCTs hints at, these marginal or 'antagonistic' virtualities that become actualized are 'corporeal' as well as 'social', 'microbiological' as well as 'political', 'pharmacological' as well as 'ethical'.[1]

The complexity of what comprises PrEP RCTs

In Chapters 2 and 4 we addressed the sheer complexity of PrEP RCTs not least as it manifests itself in 'offshore' trial sites. Especially in the last chapter we saw how this complexity, that is both human and nonhuman, is something that confronts trialists and practitioners who, in turn, attempt to 'domesticate' it by drawing on such skills as simplifying, disambiguating, itemizing, reducing and comparing. We distilled these various activities into a single term – quantification – which served to denote the use of external criteria in order to characterize an RCT, whether as a technical biomedical exercise or a bioethical endeavour. However, as we also documented in that chapter, these quantifying efforts bring with them their own specific and often unanticipated relations and dynamics. In this chapter, we pursue in more detail the struggles that scientists confront in facing up to this complexity – what we shall call 'qualification' – while they are simultaneously being drawn toward their standard forms of 'quantification'. Inevitably, we must focus on only a few examples of these struggles. However, in order to impress again the 'sheer complexity' of the trials, we revisit a sample of parameters and variables – or, in Whiteheadian terms, the prehensions – that go into the making of an RCT. These are taken from the descriptions of PrEP RCTs and PrEP by PrEP's various stakeholders.

The following list might be read as a partial compendium of the features of PrEP or PrEP RCTs that are understood within the HIV prevention field to present major challenges. Put another way, the events that we list below serve as a basis for the analysis of qualification that follows in the rest of the chapter insofar as they point to the possibility of an alternative eventuation of PrEP RCTs, bioethics and the pill.

Item 1: Disinhibition/Recalculation

For those conducting RCTs there is at a least partial recognition that the RCT will have complex effects upon the participants. In this sense, what is more or less tacitly envisaged is a participant who, in being-with new technologies (such as PrEP) that promise a possible reduction in their risk, may alter his/her otherwise safe sex practices (in both the placebo and a partially effective product arm) and, in turn, could be placed at increased risk of HIV infection. As a corollary with PrEP, there is also a concern that if it were to become available after the RCT it may reduce the perceived risk of HIV and lower condom use. Some individuals may assume that they or their sexual partners (if on PrEP) are sufficiently protected by PrEP. In sum, presumed changes in people's tacit risk calculus could significantly undermine condom use not only during the RCT, but also subsequently.

Contrary to this potential for what is referred to as 'disinhibition' (see Padian et al., 2008), there is the view that, as part of the trial, the provision of 'risk reduction counselling' along with the ready availability of prevention materials such as condoms or even male circumcision, reduces risk. Ironically, this raises some consternation. The 'unfortunate' technical side-effect of achieving lower levels of infection is that the number of infections that arise in the placebo arm will be insufficient to evidence efficacy in the treatment arm (Padian et al., 2010).[2]

Item 2: Presumption of gender and economic relations of power

Initially, much of the impetus for a biomedical prevention technology came from the Global Campaign for Microbicides (GCM) set up with a feminist intention to 'empower' women by providing them with the means to protect themselves and their partners. The aim was to provide an intervention that would not require a male sexual partner's collaboration.[3] PrEP may offer women a prevention technology that they can use without letting it be known to their partner, a partner who they may suspect has had relations with other women and may be HIV positive. However, this formulation of women is based very much on a certain conception of an individual, a conception that might well be characterized as a neoliberal autonomous subject, whereas some women may not think of, or enact, themselves in this way (see, for example, Woodsong and Karim, 2005). Rather, they may regard themselves as an extension of their male partner or as a member of a kinship network whose sexual and reproductive activities are not theirs to determine (Woodsong and Karim, 2005). In various ways, then, PrEP may enter into and potentially alter gender relations. Conversely, it may be the case that such gender or kinship (or other) relations are so entrenched that PrEP becomes something other than simply a preventative intervention. For example, by ensuring 'her' health against HIV infection and illness, a woman may retain her function as the primary carer in a family unit in a manner that is possibly, although of course not necessarily, subordinate within this set of relations.

Item 3: Physical differences between men and women

Results from trials to date suggest that there may be differences between men and women, although, as we discuss later, this is a highly convoluted picture. While the efficacy of PrEP has been established in RCTs with men who have sex with men (MSM), and there is evidence from other studies that it works in women, two large trials involving women-only participants – Fem-PrEP and VOICE discussed in Chapter 4 – have produced confounding results. At this time, the main explanation offered for disparities in results between men and women seems to be that the women participants in Fem-PrEP and VOICE have been less adherent to the dosing requirements of PrEP than in the other trials.

Item 4: Viral adaptation/waning of efficacy

One of the concerns with using antiretroviral drugs that may not give *full* protection is that a person using the drugs will become infected with HIV. In such circumstances, PrEP can be understood to morph from a prevention technology to a 'sub-optimal' therapy. The 'sub-optimal' qualifier is because, as noted briefly in Chapter 1, Tenofovir, or the combination of Tenofovir and Emtricitibane in Truvada, may not sufficiently suppress the process of viral replication during early or ongoing infection and result in the emergence of a drug resistant strain of 'the' virus (Van Damme and Szpir, 2012). In turn, this may reduce the range of treatment options and is of special concern to any country in which the drug therapy options are relatively few. A further concern is that an unknowingly newly infected person continues to take PrEP on the presumption that he or she is still HIV negative, has unprotected sex (without a condom) with a known HIV negative partner. This could lead not only to further infections but in theory at least also to infections that are potentially drug resistant (see Paxton et al., 2007:89 for an argument against this concern).

Item 5: Dosing

So far PrEP has been trialled as a pill a day intervention. It has been shown to be most efficacious when it is taken consistently on a daily basis. In the iPrEX study, infections occurred amongst those reporting inconsistent use and/or amongst those whose blood tests showed no evidence of the presence of PrEP (Grant et al., 2010). However, this account is complicated by the lack of clarity over the most suitable dosing 'tactic': thus it might be the case that taking PrEP for 24 hours, or 2 days before exposure; or immediately before and, then for a longer period after exposure, might be sufficient.

Item 6: Timeframe of trial and 'frailty'

The point of RCTs is that they generate statistical evidence of an effect. However, it is not always clear what is responsible for an effect. As noted in Chapter 4, the figures are derived at intervals that may be mapping something more than simply the number of new infections. For instance, as we noted in reference to O'Hagan et al. (2012), the cohort in the placebo arm may be subject to a selective temporal effect whereby those participants most at risk become infected early on, while those who remain uninfected continue to be so over the subsequent course of the trial, that is, they continue to be less at risk. If this pattern occurs, then the difference between the two arms of a trial reduces over time: results that might have initially indicated an efficacious intervention in the experimental arm may come to look no different to the results in the placebo arm.

Item 7: Noncompliance

For trialists one of the important measures in a trial is dosing compliance, and increasingly blood tests are used alongside self-reporting to monitor compliance. If drug levels in the blood are found to be low, this is taken as an indication of possible poor adherence even if the self-reporting indicates otherwise. However, the practice of dosing is recognized to be somewhat contingent on other factors. For instance, the women in the FEM-PrEP trial have been reported as possibly less likely to have been compliant compared to the Partners Study because they were younger, single and believed they were subject to low risk. For the women in the Partners Study who were in a relationship with a known seropositive partner, the fact that they were in a relationship was presumed to provide the incentive to dose.

Item 8: Local government and community support

All RCTs require the agreement of the government of the country in which they are being held. Considerations over whether a RCT should take place include not only the assent of a country's relevant authorities but also an assessment by trialists of that country's resources. The assessment may extend to an evaluation of how the trial itself may contribute to capacity-building in relation to the medical infrastructure. The process of realizing a RCT is, itself, lengthy and involves numerous actors who enlist support from the community, make arrangements to provide treatment for participants who become HIV-infected during a trial, organize compensation for participants who experience trial-related adverse events, and implement informed-consent procedures (see Lagakos and Gable, 2008). Taking these points together, we can see that an RCT entails a multiplicity of practical measures that have complex ramifications for the do-ability of the trial at pragmatic, ethical and epistemic levels. Indeed, in the previous chapter it was made evident that many actors may partake in how a trial eventuates, for example: research participants, activist groups, trial sponsors, international aid funding.

Item 9: Impact of testing for HIV infection prior to entry into a trial

Prior to the undertaking of a biomedical prevention trial for an intervention such as PrEP, it is necessary to make certain that the participants are HIV seronegative, that is, that they do not already have the virus. Because an HIV positive result is anticipated to be a major life-changing phenomenon, positive results are usually given in the context of counselling. But, as we saw in the preceding chapter, the revelation of HIV positive status has implications and impacts beyond the potential trial volunteer.

Item 10: Recruitment and retention

Recruitment and retention for HIV biomedical prevention RCTs – which may involve up to several thousand participants at one site or multiple sites – may be hampered by resource-poor settings with limited infrastructure and by highly mobile and diverse populations. Follow-up on completion of the RCT may take place over several years. If there is slow accrual or poor retention of trial participants, the trial may be underpowered or, according to the RCT framing, produce skewed results.

Item 11: Contexts of informed consent

Obtaining what is termed the informed consent of a research participant is a standard ethical requirement of biomedical research as with social research, yet continues to be recognized as problematic. In part, this is because informed consent is grounded in a culturally specific presumption of the autonomous individual – a presumption characteristic of the countries where sponsors and many principal investigators of RCTs reside – but not necessarily relevant to the locale of the RCT (see, for example, Woodsong et al., 2006; Woodsong and Karim, 2005). According to a study by Ruzario et al. (2012) female trial participants in regular heterosexual relationships differed in how they conceive their relationship to their partner. Some reported that 'he' should be involved in their decision to consent which suggests that they did not see themselves as the appropriate consenting subject. The general point is that while consent can be seen to serve as a marker of respect and agreement that simplifies involvement in the RCT for trialist and volunteer alike, in its practical negotiation and establishment, consent may generate a spectrum of issues which range from the process of explaining the trial and the presumption that prospective participants know the right questions to ask in order to be sure of how the trial may affect them (Mahvu et al., 2012), to the cultural inappropriateness of seeking consent in communal societies in which community representatives influence decisions about participation in activities, including research projects. Along similar lines, and in keeping with the dictates of giving consent, participants may be required by a trial to engage in practices, which may be contrary to, or conflict with, local cultural norms. The example offered by Woodsong and Karim (2005:413) is that of topical microbicide research which requires women to discontinue practices such as using vaginal drying agents. Another example is the insistence that married partners use condoms.

To be sure, the issues raised in this section comprise a very partial list, as will become apparent when additional issues are addressed below. The key point is not that the PrEP RCT is a heterogeneous event of enormous complexity – that should be obvious enough. Rather, it is that this complexity enfolds a series of virtualities. In the previous chapter, we saw how these included the attractor of what we called 'gold standard-ness'. We shall see this again, but we shall now explore how trialists themselves are aware of, and grapple with, how this gold standard-ness is emergent, a matter of laborious accomplishment, a goal always already on the brink of disintegration. But further, we shall also trace how gold standard-ness can serve as an anti-attractor that lures a very different and divergent set of prospects for the trial in question.

Three eventuations of gold standard-ness

In this section we consider the ways in which gold standard-ness emerges through, rather than is 'imposed' on, the process of a trial. So, rather than see it as an 'entity' that enters the trial event, or an external standard toward which the trial event is 'attracted', we trace how it 'becomes-with' in relation to, for instance, the complex and multiple enactments of the PrEP pill, women and men as both bodies and social actors, the trial as a technical exercise, and the ethics that putatively underpin RCTs. Inevitably, these are not always easy to disentangle; however, we have organized the discussion around three broad examples that we have labelled: RCT and Methodology, Pill (Bodies and Agency), and Ethics.

RCT and methodology

In the previous chapter we examined how the PrEP RCTs were 'singularized', not least in their guise as exemplifications of a generic–gold standard – form of testing for the efficacy of new medical interventions. We noted how external parameters of design and calculation were used in the enactment of the RCTs as a quantitative object that embodied gold standard-ness. We also mapped several of the challenges faced by various actors involved in the pursuit of gold standard-ly trials. However, we propose that the PrEP RCT can be rethought in terms of a qualitative thing which is emergent – becomes-with – in the concrete eventuation of the trial. Here the trial is not simply an event that is, primarily, clinical rather than, say, political, or economic, or cultural. Of course, scientists know full well that the trial event is all these things too. After all, they must arrange – that is, entangle themselves in – the political, economic and cultural complexities of those offshore settings in order to ensure that these trials can happen in the first place. However, these elements are usually seen as extraneous to the essence of the trial. That is, they are seen as secondary qualities to the primary ones of clinical and ethical gold standard-ness. Below, we again draw from the comprehensive guide to conducting RCTs within the HIV field edited by Lagakos and Gable (2008), in order to demonstrate how this local complexity is at once acknowledged but then addressed as a secondary quality that is 'added' to the primary quality of the rigorous – gold stardard-ly – randomized controlled trial.

We see the primary qualities set out in the following remarks:

> When planning a late-stage randomized clinical trial, investigators need to consider a number of design features, including (1) the number of subjects and duration of follow-up; (2) whether the trial will evaluate efficacy or effectiveness; (3) whether to begin with a smaller (phase 2) trial, with the understanding that a larger (phase 3) trial will follow if the results are promising...; and (4) how to choose a control group or groups. (Lagakos and Gable, 2008:69)

But these are then qualified by secondary qualities that might characterize the trials:

> A number of factors influence these choices, including the anticipated HIV incidence rate for the control group(s), the rates of product nonadherence and discontinuation owing to pregnancy and other reasons, and the rates of loss to follow-up, as well as the uncertainty surrounding these assumed rates and the resulting effect on the power of the trial. Investigators must also consider how large and long-lasting the effect of the intervention must be to be of scientific interest or public health significance. (Lagakos and Gable, 2008:69)

This complex array of contingencies, rather than being seen as integral to the trial, are factors that can be overcome such that the standardized knowledge can be sustained. This standardization is particularly prominent in a discussion of the comparability of different trial designs. Accordingly, these different designs will have the same statistical power though they will differ along a number of external parameters such as the accrual of volunteers per year, the number of years of accrual, the total participants accrued, and the duration of a trial in years (see discussion in Chapter 4). At the same time, these parameters can be realized if the complex nexus of other factors (secondary qualities) mentioned above is properly anticipated. As the text goes on to recommend:

> Investigators should take steps to develop accurate *a priori* estimates of rates of participant accrual, HIV incidence, product discontinuation, and participant retention, and incorporate those into the sample size calculations. As a guard against inaccurate estimates, investigators should consider using an 'events-driven' approach. That is, investigators would analyze study results when the prespecified number of enrolled subjects have become HIV infected, rather than at prespecified calendar times. (Lagakos and Gable, 2008:75)

However, 'to develop accurate *a priori* estimates of....' assumes two things that from our analytic perspective seem peculiar. Firstly, it seems to be assumed that the process through which it is possible 'to develop accurate *a priori* estimates of....' has no impact on the prospective volunteer populations. This is itself a matter of empirical query. More importantly, it seems to be assumed that the intervention itself does not impact upon product discontinuation, HIV incidence, participant retention and so on. Clearly, in this text there is an effort to take into account the complexity of the trial event. But rather than see the RCT as emerging from that complexity, and thus orienting one's questions to the specificity of that RCT event, there is a systematic attempt to excise this complexity so that the (gold) standardized quality of the RCT can be sustained (not least across different trial designs).

A similar pattern can be found in the following quote from a paper that traced HIV acquisition in three different groups of women:

> In this evaluation of risk factors for HIV acquisition, important differences were seen in drivers of HIV incidence at the 3 study locations. Results from this analysis imply that targeted HIV programming could have a large impact on incident HIV infection in women, and

that the most effective approach will likely vary based on knowledge of the local situation/epidemiology. (Mavedzenge et al., 2011:98)

While this is certainly an advance insofar as a local sensibility is being advocated, it neglects the fact that the process of deriving 'risk factors' is itself partially constitutive of those factors. Thus, in asking women to report on the number of sexual partners they have had, or the incidence of sexual encounters under the influence of drugs or alcohol, it is assumed that the reporting of these will be standard across the three groups. For instance, for those groups where there were relatively low numbers of sexual partners reported, it is arguably the case that there are social norms for (let us call it) 'fidelity' part and parcel of which is the enunciation of fidelity. Conversely, where there were relatively high numbers of sexual partners, it is possible that not only is having more sexual partners accepted, so too are statements to that effect. The general point is that these groups might possibly polarize in their accounting of sexual partners – the former under-estimating, the latter over-estimating. As such, these reports are not simply representations. Even though such 'sensitive information, including sexual behavior, was collected using audio computer-assisted self-interviewing' (Mavedzenge et al., 2011:90), the presentation of such information is nevertheless performative in that it serves in the re-making of local social relations and cultural conditions. What seems to be preferable to this form of seemingly unbiased quantification (in both empirical and ontological senses) is a more extended qualitative engagement with these groups of women.

However, there are some researchers who are beginning to realize that such complexity must not be 'dealt with' (quantified) but regarded as integral to the trial or study. Below we provide an extended but particularly clear articulation of this from McGrory et al.'s report (2009) which – despite invoking, albeit with a touch of irony, a clear demarcation in the practice of laboratory science and the social (as if science is not cultural in the sense of always already bound up with the political, economic etc.) – offers an insight in the complexities of the field:

> Broadly speaking, the central message is unmistakable: In the laboratory perhaps, science can indulge its natural preferences for objectivity, political neutrality, and pristine research environments. But in the field of HIV prevention research, with its numerous sensitivities, that expectation is naïve and can invite failure. Researchers need to fully internalise that insufficient attention to political context, ethical issues, and public perception can halt a clinical trial as definitively

and quickly as negative findings at a data safety and monitoring board review. This means that prevention researchers need to do more than nod to 'social factors'. They need to think about human, social, and political issues actively and strategically at every step of the conceptualization, design, conduct, and follow-through of trials. This is especially true in resource-constrained countries where economic disparities and complex colonial histories are involved and, even more so, when issues involving sex and gender are central.

Moving beyond the basics is not easy. Securing research funding, producing credible data and negotiating peer review panels is hard enough without simultaneously introducing sociology, history, politics, and mass media management into research plans and budgets. Yet fairly or not, prevention trials seem to realistically require just that. (McGrory et al., 2009:6)

This is a promising statement because it sets the scene for an emergence of the RCT that is rather different from the standard account. Indeed, it opens up the prospect for posing more interesting questions. Rather than asking how we might estimate complicating factors in order to ensure the gold standardized power of an RCT, new questions begin to emerge such as what disciplines need to inform such a process of deriving credible and robust data. The RCT thus becomes – emerges as – an occasion for drawing together an interdisciplinary range of perspectives and procedures. In the process, gold standard-ness itself shifts from signifying a certain type of focused rigour, to addressing the production of credible and robust knowledge in highly complex trial settings.

Pill (bodies and agency)

In contrast to the last chapter's focus on accounts that enact the PrEP pill as a singularized quantitative object impacting upon the body, here we focus on the ways that scientists have attempted to grasp the way that the pill has emerged through the trial. To be sure, even as a quantitative object the pill's effects are not simple but vary across bodies. After all, that is what the various statistical tests that apply to RCTs are designed to access: variation needs to be 'dealt with' in order to establish statistical significance. In the process, measures of efficacy are set against particular external parameters that ensure the singularity of the pill. Yet, to understand the pill that enters the event of the trial in this way it is not only necessarily to neglect or downplay the pill's complicating role, but to compromise the complexity of its eventuation within the trial – a complexity in which it is, itself, transformed through its intra-actions with other entities within the trial event.

Again, scientists certainly acknowledge this complexity, at least in part. For example, extensive empirical and analytic effort is directed to addressing how 'the' PrEP pill varies across, bodies, body states, body parts and formulations. The following quote amply attests to what elsewhere we have discussed as the ontological multiplicity of PrEP (see, for example, Rosengarten and Michael, 2009b). Although rather complex in its account, it draws attention to not only how the drugs work differently due to heterogeneous phenomena – for example, metabolics, genetics and so on – but that drug efficacy *and* modes of assessment of efficacy vary. Although all antiretroviral drugs can be visibilized in peripheral blood (for example, taken from the arm), the drug itself affects how well such blood can serve as a surrogate marker of penetration of relevant tissue (for example, the walls of the vagina). That is to say, the tracking of a drug in the body affects what that drug becomes – preventative or not:

> There could be differences in drug exposure because of genetics, there could be differences in drug exposure because of environment, because of dietary influences, or nutrition or malnutrition issues as well, so different populations could definitely have different exposures...The drug has to track from the blood – when taken orally – from the blood, through the tissues, and then into the cervico-vaginal fluid............And what we found is that certain drugs concentrated in the vaginal fluid, compared to blood plasma, four, five, or six-fold higher in the vaginal fluid than in blood plasma. And other drugs were much lower in the vaginal fluid than in blood plasma – 1 percent, 10 percent of what we saw in blood plasma. So the drugs themselves, the physical chemical properties of the drugs themselves, are very different, and produce very different results, depending upon which drug you're looking at. (R11)

Yet, for all its analytic sophistication, not least the recognition that the properties of various drugs emerge differently in relation to different body locales and fluids, the emphasis remains on 'the physical chemical properties of the drugs themselves'. Drugs are thus regarded as being 'in themselves', entering into a relation of 'being with' in the event of the trial, as opposed to 'becoming with' the events in which they are a part. This is not to deny that drugs have measurable effects. The problem that is being formulated here concerns how to gather accurate measures of the concentration of the drug in cervico-vaginal fluid compared with plasma. That is to say, the problem already bears the assumption that a measure *should* be generalizable or available to extrapolation when, at the same time, it is recognized that different drugs work differently. In other words, there is a resistance to precisely what the above account draws attention to: namely, the need to work *with* the generating of differences.

All we are doing here is insisting that the specificities of the elements that contribute to the redefinition of the trial event – a redefinition that grapples with the particularity of the PrEP pill's 'physical chemical properties' as they co-emerge with bodies that are social as well as physical. Put another way, the pill (now complexly 're-informed' in the process of its deployment in the trial) serves in the enactment of complex social boundaries and social bodies. The following extract, provides a vivid picture of this, especially in relation to the position of women:

> We're certainly in a situation in which this [PrEP] could be the ultimate female controlled method, because if it doesn't have to be applied genitally, then there shouldn't be any reason that the woman's partner would know that they're doing anything for prevention. It shouldn't in any way interfere with sexual activity. That can still go on in whatever way the couple chooses for that to go on…But for women where they may have…women in situations in which they don't feel that they have the ability to make open decisions with their partners…that we also want to be careful that it's not exploited in some way. For instance, a study of vaccine attitudes in the Dominican Republic found, when they interviewed sex workers, the female sex workers were excited about vaccine research, but they also said: 'We're concerned that if we find a safe and effective vaccine, that men will use that as a reason to…to not use condoms, and we won't be able to get them to use condoms, because they'll say, "No, you're going to get the vaccine", or "You've gotten the vaccine, and therefore I refuse to use condoms"'. And what the men said was, 'A vaccine would be great, because then I'll refuse to use condoms', and 'I can have as many partners as I want'. So you wouldn't want there to be a situation like that with PrEP either. I think that we should never assume that any of these strategies is going to be a hundred per cent safe and effective, and I think we're going to still have to find ways to protect women and men from exposures that they don't want to have. (R04)

This statement clearly evokes previous mention of 'disinhibition' – the likelihood that a prevention intervention may counteract or lessen existing preventive sexual practices so that risk of infection increases. Here, the pill be can be read as 'becoming with' human bodies and agencies in a process of disinhibition in which it is partially effective. And yet, the more typical account enacts a 'neutral' or 'good' PrEP as subject to the vagaries of human agency, specifically, to people's incapacity to enact the pills 'correctly' (Rosengarten, 2009:9).

By contrast, we can conceptualize the eventuation of the trial in rather different terms. For instance, PrEP may indeed serve to reduce the reliance by some women on a male partner's condom use. But PrEP may also feed into men's modes of thinking and acting, which subsequently affect women becoming embodied in their own modes of thinking and acting. In some respects, this is not dissimilar to the way that the consequences of hormonal contraception are borne by women's bodies. As such, PrEP might well at once reinforce and reconfigure, local social and cultural relations typified by specific forms of sex differentiation. For instance, PrEP might address the higher risk and rates of HIV infection for women but replace these with embodied risk of drug side-effects that requires medical surveillance, manifests *actual* drug side-effects, places women under demands of dosing adherence and, depending on levels of embodied 'partial effectiveness', continues to expose women to rates of HIV (albeit that these are likely to be reduced). The broader point is that the relationship between PrEP and women is but one illustration of how PrEP comes to manifest multiple functionalities that emerge in its relations with its numerous users. As should be clear, as PrEP becomes-with, these functionalities extend well beyond the medical and the clinical frame of safe and effective HIV prevention into the diverse complexities of sociomaterial life.

In sum, the pill is embroiled in an event that overspills the confines of 'physical chemical properties' and the affected physical body states, body types and body parts that the pill is, itself, involved in demarcating (in the above case, this is the eventuation of particular embodied women). This reformulation also reconfigures the pill as an object of expectation and a marker of future events. The expectation is not about refining an account of its effects in order to effect its refinement, that is, finding solutions for its efficacious operation. It is not in an event of being-with in which the pill combines with bodies while each retain their identities (as measured against external parameters). Rather, the pill is a qualitative thing emerging *with* its parameters, its bodies and their parameters (which now, as we have seen, incorporate the social dynamics of gendering).

If what PrEP 'is' emerges in complex ways within individual RCTs, when RCTs are taken together this complexity reaches dizzying heights. We return to the series of studies discussed in Chapter 4 and retrace a sequence of reports about various RCTs, each report documenting more or less dramatic differences in results, and more or less divergent explanations for those differences. By revisiting some of the RCT findings, we see how readily an explanation is sought in a bifurcated notion of 'woman' that maps onto the biological or 'body' versus the social or behavioural 'subject' distinction. Eventuated through this is a body that is too complex or a subject that is overly recalcitrant – both of which are the undoing of what would otherwise, seemingly, be a singular efficacious pill-object.

To recall, reported findings from PrEP RCTs in 2011 and 2012 provided divergent results in relation to women. Not surprisingly, the data from the RCTs involving women was scrutinized for a causal explanation for the failure to show efficacy. As we have already noted in Chapter 4, reports from the Fem-PrEP RCT sponsor, FHI (Family Health International), have suggested that the women may have practised poor dosing adherence (in contrast with men who have sex with men) or there may be an actual lack of effect of the product among women. Poor dosing adherence was the most favoured explanation on the basis that biochemical evidence showed that the drugs in PrEP do penetrate the female genital tract, that is, that they can work in women. This was underlined by evidence from the Partner's study (and a smaller RCT in Botswana).[4] However if, as analyses of drug levels in the blood of the women suggest, the women were not taking the pill as required, and equal numbers as those in the placebo arm became HIV infected, then this would seem to point to a more important consideration. Rather than seek a causal explanation for the absence of drug efficacy which diverts attention from the long-term goal of achieving HIV prevention, it seems crucial that some attempt be made to better understand the complex relations that were eventuated in this trial, relations that might well extend far beyond the limits of this particular trial. Additionally, as we mentioned above, it was also reported that there was an 'unexpected' higher number of pregnancies in the Truvada arm compared to the placebo arm in the Fem-PrEP trial.[5] Commentaries on the trial have not focused on the possible significance of this co-affective and possibly risk-enhancing dimension to HIV risk in women (Gray et al., 2005). Moreover they have failed to fully reflect on the possible differential ways in which pregnancy, contraception, HIV infection, 'poor' and 'good' adherence co-emerge along with differential understandings about, and negotiations of, risk of infection, and risk of, or desire for, pregnancy.

Despite the important need to better understand and, indeed, conceptualize what took place, as we have noted so far the explanation most frequently offered is that women in the FEM-PrEP trial were less adherent.

This amounted to an explanation in terms of a failure on the part of the women in the Fem-PrEP trial. This was made especially clear in an article 'A tale of two trials: how adherence is everything in PrEP':

> Participants in the [the Fem-PrEP] study said they took their pills 95 percent of the time and adherence as measured by pill count was 85 percent. However when drug levels of tenofovir and FTC were measured in the blood of women assigned to Truvada, the investigators found that less than 50 percent of the women who should have been taking the drug had actually done so in the last 12 days, and less than 40 percent within the last 48 hours. (AIDSMAP, 2012)

However the article also offers a glimpse of other factors. It states that both the Partners PrEP Study and Fem-PrEP found the only side-effect that was measurably different between drug and placebo was nausea and vomiting but notes:

> In Partners PrEP Truvada was associated with a modest increase in gastro-intestinal symptoms in the first month and in FEM-PrEP the rates were also significantly higher. Whether this is enough to deter participants from continuing their pills who are not strongly motivated needs further research. (AIDSMAP, 2012)

As mentioned above, the visceral and social 'prominence' of these side-effects might be shaped by the extent to which participants are 'strongly motivated' to continue with PrEP. This becomes clearer when, later in the same article, the question of differences in adherence is addressed by the respective Principal Investigators of the Partners PrEP and Fem-PrEP trials, one trial which displayed high adherence to PrEP use and one that did not. Jared Baeten, Principal Investigator for Partners PrEP is reported as stating that the men and women in the Partners Study defined themselves as being in a stable relationship and that partners would have encouraged the trial participants to take their pills. A qualitative study is noted by Baeten to have confirmed that 'many participants saw PrEP as an opportunity to preserve their relationship despite the strain imposed by different HIV status.' In contrast, we learn from Lut Van Damme, Principal Investigator of Fem-PrEP that Fem-PrEP enrolled a cohort of women who were much younger than the women enrolled to the other studies (including Partners PrEP but also VOICE); and these younger women were also known to have relatively high levels of sexually transmitted infections. She is quoted as stating:

Initial qualitative surveys had shown that many did not believe themselves to be at high risk of HIV, despite high incidence in their community. There was also a high pregnancy rate in the study despite reported high levels of oral contraceptive use, showing that low adherence to medications was not restricted to Truvada. There was no evidence that participants were sharing their pills with others and, contrary to what the data initially suggested, the pregnancy rate was no higher in women taking PrEP, ruling out theories that inter-actions between the PrEP drugs and the menstrual cycle may have made women more vulnerable to HIV. (AIDSMAP, 2012)

So, although the complexity of adherence is partially addressed in the above statements, it tends to remain an external parameter of the trial. This is made especially apparent at the close of the article by Sharon Hillier of MTN (Microbicides Trial Network): 'PrEP is very, very effective if you use it very, very well.'

In all, the approach to PrEP is somewhat reminiscent of Wynne's (1989) analysis of the expert authorities accounting for the toxicological impact of pesticides amongst farm workers: as long as the instructions were followed, then there was no risk. Wynne suggests that this reflects a sociological naiveté in relation to the complex conditions to be found on a farm where 'following the instructions' is not always practicable. At a meta-level, this is of course sociologically sophisticated insofar as it transfers responsibility from manufacturers to users. Adherence to dosing in women volunteers, or adherence to instructions in farm workers, remain external parameters that can be interjected into an event rather than seen to be emergent from the event itself where 'adherence' is less a problem in need of a solution, and more a lure for creatively rethinking the 'nature' of the trial or farming event.

Specifically, our point is that adherence emerges in the confluence and co-emergence of PrEP, bodies and agency in the specific eventuation of the trials. In the Partners trial, PrEP comprises an additional medi-ator through which to sustain relationships within HIV status diver-gent couples. PrEP is another relationality – that is, a resource – that enables the exercise of particular sorts of agency and the enactment of particular sorts of bodies within the eventuation of particular fraught sexual relationships. By contrast, in the Fem-PrEP trial, PrEP becomes a different sort of resource. Contrary to the statement above that partici-pants 'did not believe themselves to be at high risk of HIV', the obser-vation that the taking of contraceptive pills was lax, suggests a culture in which sexual practices entailed comparatively high risk-taking or risk-indifference. PrEP is thus not subject to non-adherence, but becomes a resource for the continued enactment of particular 'risky' bodies and selves. The corollary notions of adherence and non adherence – while they can afford some access the heterogeneity and complexity of populations – do not address how an intervention such as PrEP becomes-with in the specific eventuations of the trial (nor how the RCT itself is transformed). On this score, in both the Fem-PrEP and Partners RCTs, PrEP has indeed been used, as Hillier put it in the quote above, 'very, very well' though to the rather different ends of eventuating widely divergent sociomaterial relationships.

Ethics

In the previous chapter, we considered the ways in which ethics were subject to gold standard-ness. We noted how external criteria were mobilized in the form of the two ethicalities of RCTs, a technical ethicality in which the trials must be designed in such a way as to make them valuable for the larger at-risk population, and a local or social ethicality where the rights of local volunteer population were upheld. We argued that these are not always consonant. In the present chapter, we begin to trace how researchers are grappling with the complexity of these ethics and, in particular, with how these ethics can be treated as emergent or 'becoming-with' in the eventuation of trials. However, as we simply mention, and elaborate in the next, this entails what we might call topological relationalities.

Our first example is a WHO/UNAIDS (2004) report '*Treating people with intercurrent infection in HIV prevention trials*' in which the provision of antiretroviral drugs for people who seroconvert over the course of a trial was justified on the basis that 'the occurrence of HIV infection is required in order to demonstrate the efficacy of the prevention intervention' (WHO/UNAIDS, 2004:4). Later, the report complicates this commitment by raising a series of questions about, for instance, what level of care should be provided (care equivalent to that available at the trial location, or in sponsor country medicine – these are often vastly different), who is responsible, and whether a partner should receive antiretrovirals at levels comparable with those who were enrolled in the trial (2004:4). Ultimately, we are left with a sense that, although the moral commitment to trial participants is clearly evident, the complex practicalities prevent the aim of an internationally standardized ethical commitment from being realized. In sum, it seems that scientific researchers find themselves facing what may appear as an ethical quandary in which they must collectively struggle to know how to act ethically in a setting marked by asymmetrical relations between researchers and volunteers, and the local poverty of clinical resources.

This ethical quandary is further complicated by the implications of this contrast between what is medically available in the home country of the sponsors and the lead researchers, and relatively impoverished provision available to trial participants in a developing country. That is to say, trial-incurred needs (for example, HIV infection developed in the course of participating in an RCT) may place yet more pressure on what are already inadequate or stretched familial, local and national resources. Perhaps most indicative of how the vulnerability important to HIV RCTs may be compounded is the issue of 'disinhibition' mentioned at several points above. As we have noted, a trial bearing the promise of an effective intervention has the potential to lead to more unsafe practice resulting in increases in infection (AVAC, 2008). The unhappy irony is that this reinforces the impoverished conditions associated with HIV vulnerability, which also reinforces that site's suitability for RCTs. The tragedy is that this could mean an increase in the number of people with infections, people who have limited or no access to the drugs for treatment.

So, although increasingly researchers are committed to ensuring the provision of antiretroviral access (and this commitment is made more possible as treatment access improves in middle and some low income countries), international agencies such as WHO and UNAIDS have demonstrated, at best, ambivalence toward researchers' immediate obligations of care to their research subjects. The ambivalence is compounded by the way that bioethics entails the externalization of much of what is involved in the day-to-day lives of the participants. It is first and foremost concerned with such issues as participant consent, the weighing of benefit over risk, and reciprocity in the form of later access to the intervention under trial. Even, where the bioethical horizon is expanded in relation to a specific trial site or a particular sample of participants, this can nevertheless be treated by trialists as a problem for the conduct of a trial. Let us return to a quote (referred to in Chapter 4) from a leading (publicly funded) scientist writing on the problematics of providing trial participants with the best standard of prevention:

> *To comply with ethical guidelines, we have reduced our ability to assess new prevention methods* [our emphasis] by comparing them to the best available prevention standards of care (for example, limitless sexually transmitted infection treatment; frequent, individualised, and expensive

condom counselling). Such strategies are not representative of the standard of typical prevention services in the community and are not sustainable after completion of the trial. (Padian et al., 2008:593)

As noted above, it is apparent in this statement that ethics are seen as a potential hindrance to accomplishing a statistically significant outcome through the achievement of a sufficiently substantial number of HIV infections. It is also apparent that prevention counselling, referred to as 'expensive', is an obstruction to the gold standard of the trial. But even more thought-provoking is the way in which the ethicality of an RCT should be judged against the (typically impoverished) local prevention services as opposed to those that exist in the trial's sponsoring country. In other words, the ethical guidelines enacted in the context of an 'offshore trial' are seen as over-constraining because they are likely to limit infections due to comprehensive prevention counselling, provision of condoms and possibly treatment of sexually transmitted infections that may enhance HIV vulnerability.

Padian et al.'s (2008) concern that such services are not sustainable after the RCT, underscores the difference between the country of the trial sponsor and the location of the 'offshore' trial. Indeed, as we have remarked, it is this difference in prevention standards of care that makes the 'offshore' trial location attractive. There is, in sum, a privileging of the goal of achieving a biomedical prevention technology over the goal of prevention *per se*. This can also be re-framed in terms of dual local and scientific ethicalities: local ethics that yield benefits to trial participants are a cost to the sponsoring biomedical institutions who, were they to financially support treatment after the trial, would have fewer resources to devote to RCTs elsewhere.

So, in the commentaries of UNAIDS and Padian et al. (2011) there are at once hints of an acknowledgement of, but also a withdrawal from, the complexities of bioethics as enacted in relation to PrEP RCTs. For instance, Padian et al. suggest an alternative design – a 'stepped wedge randomised trial design' – where the intervention is rolled out to participants (whether individuals or groups) sequentially, that is over a series of time periods. They go on to explain:

The fundamental premise underlying randomized approaches to implementation is to concentrate implementation in a few sites (preferably selected randomly) and then to phase in other sites over time (for example, a 'stepped wedge'). This approach is in contrast to simultaneous implementation across many sites and districts and capitalizes on the logistic and fiscal realities that usually make a wide-spread simultaneous implementation approach difficult. Because study locations are randomized based on time, sites that at first do not receive the program initially serve as a comparison; however, all eligible sites eventually receive the program, ensuring equity. (2011:201)

Now, this might be a technical solution to the ethical issues that arise with the use of a parallel placebo arm for an intervention that is regarded beneficial. Eventually all participants receive the intervention. But, again, there is an application of external parameters here. Although so far we have focussed on 'offshore trials' in low and middle income countries with limited resources, a curious ethical dilemma emerges by setting up a control group 'in waiting'. If, for instance, an individual in the control group believes s/he has been exposed to the virus, a question arises over whether this individual should have immediate access to PEP (post-exposure prophylaxis). If the country context is such that the PEP is already available then it cannot be refused and must be considered part of the trial's standard of care. However, if the country locale does not already make PEP available, should individuals in the control group who report likely exposure to HIV within the estimated window period for PEP to be effective (within 72 hours of exposure) be prescribed PrEP drugs as a form of PEP? Given the drugs are understood as likely but not guaranteed to prevent infection after exposure, it could be argued that by not offering them, the trialists are prioritizing the conditions of the trial not the 'needs' of the individual.

Throughout our discussion we have sought to recognize the efforts made to grapple with the ethical complexities of RCTs, while also showing that in these efforts there seems to be a recourse to forms of standardization that are, ironically, generative of new problems. Having noted this, we now turn to an example where the heterogeneous complexities of a trial event are addressed in detail. Again, we return to an example mentioned in Chapter 4, the trial of PrEP amongst Injection Drug Users (IDU) in Bangkok sponsored by the US Centers for Disease Control and Prevention (CDC) and conducted in partnership with the Thailand Ministry of Public Health and Gilead Sciences who provided pharmaceutical support. Here we consider a letter published on the internet by a range of NGOs, such as the Thai AIDS Treatment Action Group (TTAG), the Thai Drug Users' Network (TDN), the Thai NGO Coalition on AIDS (TNCA), and the Center for AIDS Rights (CAR) that was sent to the key medical actors responsible for the trial (TTAG et al., 2004).

While the letter expresses general support for the 'Study of the Safety and Efficacy of Daily Tenofovir to Prevent HIV Infection Among Injection Drug Users in Bangkok, Thailand' a nexus of ethical concerns is raised. This includes the fact that no clean needles and syringes would be provided by the RCT (which as the best means of preventing HIV spread amongst IDU, would parallel the provision of condoms for trials focused on the sexual transmission of HIV). The authors note that this is particularly ethically problematic because the control arm involves a placebo. Moreover, they note that this target group is highly susceptible to local Thai government victimization as well as being deprived of what elsewhere would be considered basic facilities and resources. As the authors of the letter put it:

> We are concerned you have chosen a highly underserved, criminalized, and exploited group whose safety and best interests you are not in a position to protect, as required by the Declaration of Helsinki and other international ethical standards.

These difficulties faced by the trial scientists – who, it is claimed are not in a position to protect their research subjects – extended, and continues to extend, beyond ensuring the 'quality of referrals, support, treatment and care that the trial participants will receive'. Besides the overt violence against injecting drug users, it was noted that ensuring participant consent has been freely given would be difficult. Volunteers recruited from methadone clinics could, the letter went on to state: 'feel coerced into enrolling in your trial if they feel the services they receive may otherwise be compromised'.

These concerns, along with other criticisms, point to the design of this PrEP RCT as ethically deeply flawed. The flaw is further contextualized or, perhaps more aptly, inscribed in relation to a 'deepest concern...that no IDU or AIDS NGO community representatives have been involved from the outset on any official committee to discuss all aspects of the trial', not least before it has reached the upstream ethical committee stage. Although later a consultation process did take place, as we write, the design issues of the trial raised in the letter continue to apply. The critical commentary in the letter suggests that the ethicality of the trial should have been realized across different actors; most obviously, in relation to the letter, these actors would minimally include the trial scientists, volunteers' NGO representatives *and* new needles and syringes.

So, although the controversy surrounding these early PrEP RCTs can readily be seen to be well-founded, we see the articulation falls short of an effective challenge to the problematic nature of the RCT. What is proposed by those objecting to the RCTs is that an ethics appropriate to a particular event needs to draw on those various actors who have a direct investment or interest in that event. However, it can be argued that the international HIV research community believes it has solved the ethical problem of RCTs by providing guidelines for volunteer community participation. Not long after the international consultations by IAS and by UNAIDS, that aimed to account for the controversy in Cambodian and Cameroon and over Bangkok trial with injecting drug users, UNAIDS commissioned AVAC to prepare guidelines for undertaking biomedical HIV prevention trials entitled 'Good Participatory Practice' (2011). The document is rigorous in its attempt to ensure that a broad group of stakeholders and, most notably, affected HIV communities in low and middle income countries targeted for HIV RCTs, have a say in identifying areas of concern. Moreover, the report argues that RCTs be adequately resourced to take into account, and where possible to address, such concerns. As an illustration of this approach to ensuring ethical RCTs, we cite one pertinent section of the report:

> Community stakeholders can provide the best information on how to design socially and culturally acceptable strategies for recruitment, screening, enrolment, follow-up, and exit. Community stakeholders included in the process of developing these strategies can play an important role in identifying and mitigating trial-related stigma, misconceptions, or miscommunication. (2011:59)

In the present case, by pulling in a variety of actors, and even when drawing upon globalizing (see Chapter 6) ethical and moral principles such as those embodied in the Declaration of Helsinki, and affirmed by the World Medical Association and by the authors of the above cited letter, it is presumed that an ethics better suited to the specificity of the trial might emerge. However – and not withstanding our note that the opposition to the RCT was insufficient to bring about a thorough interrogation – even if it is unclear how exactly this might take place, the RCT now emerges as an occasion for thinking about who can have voice in the design of a trial. Indeed, it would even appear that there are hints here of an emerging shift in what the gold standard-ness of an RCT can be (see below).

RCT as 'anti-attractor': The prospect of something other

In this section we turn to address how trials are also events which are generative of the unexpected and the novel. That is to say, over and above the ways in which the processuality of the trial means that the RCT emerges shorn of its standard 'gold standard-ness', we explore how the openness of the trial points to a prospect or virtuality in which the event becomes something other than an RCT, or even a trial. As such, we can suggest that the abstraction of gold standard-ness serves as a sort of 'anti-attractor' that 'repels' the event toward other attractors (or external objects), which the event might take in (prehend) – attractors which might embody different ethical, political or epistemic framings.

We will begin with the example of the early PrEP trials and the controversy that arose with them. We follow by revisiting some of the material presented above with a view to deriving hints of the RCTs' potentially emerging prospects.

As we discussed in Chapter 4, the early PrEP trials generated considerable opposition. This opposition was expressed through protests both at the July 2004 XV International AIDS Society Conference in Bangkok attended by over 12,000 delegates, and in the countries where the trials were to be undertaken. The protest at the AIDS Conference attracted international media attention, particularly because of the manner in which it was staged, outside the booth of Gilead Sciences which produces the drugs used in PrEP, (Mills et al., 2005; Singh and Mills, 2005). Placards proclaimed 'Sex workers infected by Gilead'. The aim was to make it known to the conference that 960 Cambodian female sex workers were to be used as experimental subjects for PrEP RCTs. There were also protests held in Cambodia. The claims at the core of the protest were that the trial failed to provide sufficient translated information, and that care for those injured through adverse events (including provision of ARVs for those who became HIV infected while enrolled in the trial) was uncertain. Amongst the material issued by the activist groups was the following statement by Yunang Soma, head of Cambodian sex workers union:

> If they [the trial organisers] are so sure this drug is safe why don't they send their own sisters and daughters to test it? They have a lot more money than sex workers and have protection if the drug makes them sick. Also if it was their sisters and daughters they would be a lot more honest about the risks and side effects. (WNU, 2004)[6]

Now, it is certainly possible to counter the protestors' claims as being misinformed, that their arguments were based on incorrect reports in the media (Mills et al., 2005:4). For instance, it turned out that the pharmaceutical manufacturer, Gilead Sciences, was not actually directly involved in the trials and simply provided the drugs and placebo for all

PrEP trials at cost; information materials were translated into the Khmer language; and an independent data safety monitoring board, with representation from Cambodia as well as from the NIH (US National Institutes of Health), would have regularly monitored the safety data accumulated over the course of the trial (Page-Shafer et al., 2005:1501). So, even if in its specificities the protestors' statements were inaccurate and unfair, they nevertheless point to the ways in which a form of singularized bioethics focused on quantitative ethical objects, along with the quantitative objects mobilized by the RCTs and PrEP enact a particular, delimited version of the event of the trial.

The statement by Soma for WNU, quoted above, can be read as evoking the sort of uneasiness felt by many laypeople and local communities faced with the operations of biomedicine (or of technoscience more generally). Here, the form, as much as the content, of expert pronouncements (that is, the apparent certainty of expert statements) is often at odds with the contingencies experienced or perceived by local people (see, for example, Wynne, 1996; Irwin, 1996; Irwin and Michael, 2003). More specifically in the present context, it points to the asymmetrical global circumstances that underpin 'offshore trials' and the local exigencies faced by their experimental subjects. As Petryna (2007) notes in a discussion of commercial pharmaceutical research, the local desire for otherwise unavailable medicines and care may result in trials gaining government acceptance even though regulatory processes are uncertain.

Beyond this, the event of the trial becomes an agonistic occasion: a different framing of bioethics emerges. Instead of accompanying RCTs as they travel the world, serially assessing and ensuring their (demarcated) ethical status, bioethics could attend to the very process of travel. As such bioethics rather than 'solving' the particular ethical issues that arise with particular RCTs, becomes generative of more interesting problems: wrested from the hands of a professional elite, it can, for illustration, pose questions about the ethical status of offshore-ness in its various manifestations, or whether the resources that flow into the enterprise of RCTs are better routed toward lower tech, higher reliability, potentially more effective, interventions (such as the provision of condoms or clean needles). Here a different attractor comes into view – one focused less on the trialling of a drug, and more concerned with the immediate exigencies of at-risk communities.

Let us revisit the protest mentioned above, and take this together with the discussion in the 'Ethics' section of this chapter. We can re-consider those protests and proposals, and especially activist (and practitioner) recommendations for volunteer community participation. These can be placed in relation to recent ways of thinking about the heterogeneous processes by which scientific knowledge is generated. Increasingly, many types of scientific knowledge are regarded as complex, uncertain and contingent insofar as they necessarily entail social dimensions: social activity might be part of the phenomenon under study or social elements impact crucially on the measurement and modelling of the phenomena in question (for example, global climate change and its modelling or, in the present case, the rate of HIV infection). Accordingly, the knowledge produced by this post-normal (Funtowitz and Ravetz, 1993) or Mode II (Nowotny et al., 2001) science can no longer remain the preserve of scientific institutions alone. The voice of lay or public actors is increasingly seen to be vital to the production of robust scientific knowledge and numerous authors have attempted to develop mechanisms by which lay public participation can be enabled. Promising candidates for addressing such processes of engagement include, for example, Callon et al.'s (2001) notion of hybrid forums, or Stengers' (2005) concept of cosmopolitics, or Irwin and Michael's (2003) analysis of ethno-epistemic assemblages. Crucially, in all three cases, there is an attempt to conceptualize how in the encounter between various actors that might include both 'expert' and 'lay' drawn from scientific, ethical, economic or community domains, there is a prospect of becoming-with wherein the identities of the various participants shift in relation to one another. As this happens, then the issue at stake also potentially changes as the participants who have entered into the process have themselves changed and what once was central or definitive now no longer appears so, and is replaced by a reformulation of that issue – a reformulation that might also entail inventive problem-making.

Following on from the above, we can apply this sensibility to the proposal set out in the letter regarding the CDC IDU trial in Bangkok and to the recommendations of community involvement made by the HIV community. To be sure these are to be welcomed; however, we also need to ask the extent to which such 'events of discussion' can indeed incorporate 'becoming-with' in the sense that there is a possibility of mutual change between both trial scientists and community representatives and members (who, as we have seen, do not always get it 'technically right'). The 'attractor' for the trial event now concerns, amongst other things, the nature of heterogeneous and open decision-making. To re-pose the question of the trial in an interesting way is to address the circumstances under which sponsors, scientists, activists and volunteers can all mutually change – become-with – in the process of determining whether and how an interesting and relevant event – which may incorporate a trial – proceeds.

Even so, this needs to be complexified still further. Above, we noted that McGrory et al. (2009) argue for a heightened interdisciplinarity to deal with the enormous complexities of running offshore RCTs. And yet, we might also ask what does this do to trials themselves? For instance, we can pose the following question. Within such trial eventuations, what comprises 'data', let alone credible data, when one thinks 'about human, social, and political issues actively and strategically at every step of the conceptualization, design, conduct, and follow-through of trials' as McGrory et al. (2009:6) put it? And we can also ask: What constitutes evidence of efficacy and effectiveness when, to quote McGrory et al. (2009:6) again 'sociology, history, politics, and mass media manage-ment into research plans and budgets'? These seem to us to be the more interesting questions that can be asked about the nature of trials – or rather a new attractor emerges in relation to the trial, one for which 'data' becomes an altogether more complex, heterogeneous and vari-egated category. This maps onto the previous discussion of the politics of bringing together different actors in the eventuation of trials, for this also raises the issue that what can count as 'data' or 'evidence of effectiveness' is now something that is open to on-going heterogeneous negotiation. We shall return to this issue in Chapter 7 where we discuss how we might engage with becoming-with and the virtual in relation to the design and conduct of RCTs.

Finally, if we reconsider the section on Pill (Bodies and Agency), we can see how the RCT and PrEP together emerge not as an occasion for adherence, non-adherence, or disinhibition, but in an eventuation in which are enacted particular more or less locally responsible bodies and agencies (even if that responsibility to particular local cultural and social expectations entail medical risk-taking). Here, there emerges another prospective attractor – one where the complex 'intra-actions' of the nonhuman (specifically the PrEP pill) is taken into account. Rather than a mere neutral 'intermediary' that is inserted into the design of the trial, it co-emerges as something different along with those who use it – trial participants and practitioners alike.

Drawing on Stengers (2010), the PrEP pill can be said to speak through different spokespersons in a range of voices: minimally, trial participant, scientific and experiential. Such diversity understandably generates all sorts of uncertainties in the process of negotiating the nature of the event – an event that, as we hinted above, might well turn out to be something other than what is typically recognizable as an RCT. If we were to use the language of the gold standard, we would say that the gold standard – as an anti-attractor – applies less to the technics and ethics of an RCT, and more to mechanisms through which is enabled an open negotiation of what a PrEP trial event 'is'. Along the way, what is to count as 'data' is likely to be radically transformed as the problem for which data is derived, itself, markedly shifts.

Concluding remarks

In this chapter we have attempted to 'open up' the PrEP RCT and the PrEP pill by revisiting the complexities, heterogeneity and multiplicity enacted through the trials. Along the way, we have focused especially on the struggles faced by trialists (as well as activists and volunteers) as they have endeavoured to deal with these. This allowed us to begin to unravel how the gold standard-ness of the trials is eventuated both in practice and as a virtuality (an anti-attractor), and can thus become something other. If this sounds rather too vague, it is a partial upshot of our attempt to retain this sense of openness, to avoid specifying or, worse, prescribing an alternative virtuality. That will be up to the actors actually involved.

However, having made this point, we are not satisfied with simply pointing to a sensibility that engages with the virtual. We also want to 'resource' this virtuality concretely – to make suggestions about this virtuality and how it might be generative of new avenues of research and intervention. We do not view this initiative in relation to the clinical trials alone; rather, it is indissoluble from thinking about the virtualities of our own social scientific methodological and analytic practice. Indeed, here, the division between the conduct of the trials and their social scientific analysis can blur creatively. In Chapter 7 we address just this potentiality, discussing one possible route for the enactment of openness and the creative re-invention of the problem of PrEP RCTs and their objects, subjects and data. Before that, however, we want to embed the event of PrEP RCTs in relation to other events, more or less distant; or, put another way, we want to explore some of the possibly unexpected elements (prehensions) that – topologically – enter into the event of the PrEP RCT.

6
On Some Topologies of PrEP

Introduction

In this chapter we once again attend to the complex eventuations of PrEP RCTs but broaden our analytic horizons to situate these within an account of the relationship between globalization and localization. In other words, we look at the ways in which the specific emergence and role of abstraction in PrEP RCTs are played out as convolutions or, better, 'involutions' of globalizing and localizing processes. By drawing on the idea of involutions, in which the global emerges out of the local and vice versa, we return to the idea that PrEP RCTs are part of an assemblage that entails multiple and heterogeneous relations. Moreover, we imagine this assemblage topologically: topology, used circumspectly, seems to us to throw an inventive light on what PrEP RCTs are and can become. Most notably, topology allows us to trace how seemingly distal relations play a part in the eventuation of PrEP and clinical trials.

In the preceding chapters we have argued, not least through the juxtaposition of quantification and qualification, that the application of various external criteria such as those that ground gold standard-ness of RCTs neglect the ways in which PrEP RCTs are events in which their constitutive elements (pills, bodies, subjects, HIV, etc.) are emergent. As we shall elaborate below, topology is particularly suited to the analysis of such emergence – where, rather than drawing on external criteria of assessment or measurement, these criteria are seen to emerge from the event or assemblage itself, even where such an assemblage might include elements that seemingly belong elsewhere. On this score, we draw on another eventuation of HIV, this time in the particular form of UNAIDS's AIDS Clock, to examine additional aspects of the eventuation of PrEP RCTs.

It should be apparent that in some ways we have already been conducting a topological analysis, though mediated by such concepts as event and eventuation. What topology offers is an explicit focus on the spatiotemporal character of the relations between the abstraction of gold standard-ness and the various external criteria that are associated with this, and the emergence of bodies, HIV, people in specific PrEP RCTs.

For instance, let us turn again to the article by Padian et al. (2010) which both advocates 'gold standard RCTs' and engages with the issues that they throw up. In partial response to the difficulty of accurately assessing background community HIV incidence against which to measure HIV incidence within the trial, Padian et al. (2010) call for improved assays to detect when HIV infection has occurred in individuals. This would allow for a more accurate estimate of the incidence of HIV infection as it exists at the time of the trial's implementation. Improved HIV testing technologies are said potentially to 'reduce trial costs by providing a more accurate basis for sample size calculations and assisting in the more reliable selection of populations with sufficiently high HIV incidence to permit trials of shorter duration' (2010:631). The same authors also note that in the protracted delay between designing and undertaking a trial – potentially as long as a decade – the local epidemic may be affected by new interventions or changes in what they refer to as 'the epidemic phase'.

Evidently there is a keen awareness of the complex relations entailed in these measures of HIV infection and the authors advocate a continuing assessment of trialists' own 'original assumptions' (Padian et al., 2010:632). The manner by which such assumptions are to be on-goingly assessed, however, rests on a singular space-time calibration. To explicate: insofar as trialists focus on HIV incidence *per se* in order to design a trial (and even though there is clear concern that a trial might be out of date at the time of implementation because of changes in HIV incidence), HIV incidence remains the abiding criterion. This is an external criterion whose shifting value affects whether a trial is useful or otherwise: it serves to calibrate the spaces and times of the design of the trial against the times and spaces of its implementation. By comparison, our argument is that such a comparison is better understood through emerging criteria that might incorporate, for instance, availability of other drugs, or changes in local healthcare provision. In this case, the topological operation of 'homeomorphism' might usefully apply: as such, by emphasizing or de-emphasizing certain characteristics, objects (or events) that initially appear very different are rendered similar. The point for the case of PrEP RCTs is that a topological analysis of events (for example, RCTs, ethical evaluations) and things (pills, bodies) will alert us to the ways that some of these are homomorphically brought together within the same set or category (thus enabling comparability and even combinability), while others are excluded.

In what is to follow, we begin with a brief introduction to a version of topological analysis that seems to us to have particular heuristic merit in further coming to grips with the complexities of the PrEP case. We then apply this, initially to the AIDS Clock and, then, to PrEP RCTs and their ethics. To the extent that both of these can be regarded as 'globalizing' – extending their reach globally – we draw out some of the 'topological tensions' that bedevil them. We then go on to consider the topological trajectories of PrEP as it takes on three guises – as medium, as product and as affect. The aim here to is explore how PrEP, itself, operates (and is operated upon) in varying ways to produce differences and similarities across populations and practitioners, times and spaces, medical interventions and affective tactics. We finish by topologizing our own topological efforts by topologically situating our social scientific work in relation to that of a literary theorist.

Event, assemblage and topology

Earlier in this book, we noted that for the purposes of analysing PrEP RCTs, the PrEP pill and bioethics, we preferred to use the notions of event and eventuation over the concept of assemblage. This preference was partly based on the view that the English translation 'assemblage' failed to fully capture the dynamism associated with the original French term used by Deleuze and Guattari, namely 'agencement' which, as Phillips (2006) notes, was closely associated with the concept of event. In our view, and in light of the writings of such authors as Whitehead, Deleuze, Stengers and Fraser, event and eventuation allowed us to explore the temporal, prospective dimensions of PrEP RCTs – to engage with the ways in which RCTs were at once locally emergent and drawn toward the abstractions of gold standard-ness.

Here, we return to assemblage precisely because it better connotes the complex spatiality of PrEP RCT events. Of course, we have touched on this before in looking at the way that the trial events entailed elements drawn from distant parts of the world. However, our main emphasis was on how these trial events were partly comprised through elements which served to standardize or stabilize those events, or rendered them open and emergent. In other words, we focused on their 'temporalization'. By contrast, in this chapter we want to pay particular attention to

the spatialization of the PrEP trial event – the way that in the eventuation of the trial, divergent spaces can be 'brought together' (concresced)
or, rather, that spaces that are seemingly distant are within the particular eventuations of PrEP trials rendered close together (and, as we have
already hinted, this applies no less to ostensibly distant *categories*).

Needless to say, an assemblage is characterized by the heterogeneity
of its constitutive elements – a characteristic which it shares with the
'event' and with several approaches within Science and Technology
Studies, notably Actor-Network Theory. In broad terms this heterogeneity covers both content and expression. By 'content' Deleuze and
Guattari (1988:88) refer to the 'machinic' composed 'of bodies, actions
and passions, an intermingling of bodies reacting to one another'. By
contrast, 'expression' implies 'a collective assemblage of enunciation,
of acts and statements, of incorporeal transformations attributed to
bodies' (Deleuze and Guattari, 1988:88). What most concern us here
are the patternings of an assemblage. On the one hand, the elements
that make up an assemblage are territorialized insofar as they are organized in particular patterns and through particular routines. They display
a root-like quality in that there are (categories of) elements organized
in distinct linear relation to one another. For instance, in some assemblages science is enacted in opposition to 'non-scientific' actors such as
publics: in this schema, knowledge moves linearly from the former to
the latter (see Irwin and Michael, 2003). Another rootish assemblage is
the version of evolution in which species are organized in lineages that
reflect how sexual reproduction and natural selection lead to a linear
emergence of new species (see Ansell Pearson, 1999). On the other hand,
assemblages also display processes of de- (and re-) territorialization.
Here, a key metaphor is that of the rhizome: accordingly, any part of the
rhizomic assemblage can join up with any other. Thus public actors can
combine with scientific actors (and policy, media and activist ones too)
and, rather than evolution, we have involution in which genetic material moves 'anti-nuptually' across the linearities of sexual reproduction
to produce 'subterranean becomings' (Ansell Pearson, 1999:161).

Having drawn this contrast, we need to step back and reflect on the
relations between root and rhizome, territorialization and deterritorialization: as Deleuze and Guattari (1988:10) put it, 'How could move-
ments of deterritorialization and processes of reterritorialization not be
relative, always connected, caught up in one another?', after all 'there
are knots of arborescence (roots) in rhizomes, and rhizomic offshoots in
roots....The important point is that the root-tree and the canal rhizome
are not two opposed models...' (Deleuze and Guattari, 1988:20).

This non-linear connectivity is reminiscent of topological thinking. Mathematically, topology explores the 'the properties that are preserved through deformations, twistings, and stretchings of objects'[1] such that points that are distant within one schema (Euclidian) are close together in another (topological). Topology has become an increasingly popular resource for sociological and cultural thinking (see Lury et al., 2012) and there are various ways in which it has been appropriated (see, for example, Mol and Law, 1994; DeLanda, 2002; Lash and Lury, 2007). Given our present aims, we draw on three aspects of topology to inform our analysis in this chapter. Firstly, space and time are not external frameworks used to specify particular points (which might be objects or events or categories). Unlike Euclidian space where points are grasped on the basis of their position within a grid of some sort (for example, the x, y, z axes; linear clock time), for topology these frameworks emerge from the specificity of the particular event and its relations to other events. Secondly, as already noted, points which are distant can simultaneously be close together. Thirdly, while the relations between points can undergo transformation, these are open and immanent (in keeping with our notion of eventuation) rather than linear or causal.

We shall have cause to nuance our use of topology in the context of the specific empirical cases (and their relations) set out below. Suffice it to say for the moment that topology serves as a useful heuristic that can inventively illuminate the ways in which PrEP is enacted across divergent sites, while also tying those sites closer together across a number of registers – epistemically and politically, and ethically and affectively.

The AIDS Clock

We begin with what has come to be called the AIDS Clock on the website of the United Nations Population Fund (UNFPA), a device assumed by its designers to serve as a valuable (indeed value-generating) intervention by rallying support and investment to prevent the spread of HIV. In order to understand something of the intended work of the clock and how its enactment may viewed topologically, it is useful to have some background on the response to the epidemic at an international level and, notably, UNFPA itself. The organization is an international development agency that involves partnering with governments, other United Nations agencies, communities, NGOs, foundations and the private sector 'to raise awareness and mobilize the support and resources to achieve its mission' (UNFPA, 2006). The website for UNFPA states its mission is to promote 'the right of every woman, man and child to enjoy a life of health and equal opportunity' and its activities consist primarily of programmes that aim to: 'reduce poverty and to ensure that every pregnancy is wanted, every birth is safe, every young person is free of HIV/AIDS, and every girl and woman is treated with dignity and respect'.

Two features, in particular, are important for our discussion: UNFPA explicitly portrays itself as informed by the use of population data; and its activities are financed through donor contributions. In other words, population data – derived through a complex web of social, epidemiological and biomedical surveillance – directs the policy and programme activities of UNFPA but it also is understood as integral to the fund raising necessary to these activities. In all UNFPA supports programmes across about 150 countries (UNFPA, 2012).

Although our focus is not directly on funding or the economic dimensions of the epidemic, it is worth pausing here to consider what significance there might be in the difference between funds raised for biomedical trials and those for an agency such as UNFPA (particularly as UNFPA is a co-sponsor of UNAIDS which coordinates and supports an international response to the epidemic). The vision of its partner which is more specifically focused on addressing issues arising from the HIV/AIDS epidemic in contrast to UNFPA with its broader focus on poverty, sexual inequality and so on, is: 'Zero new HIV infections. Zero discrimination. Zero AIDS-related deaths'.[2] As we have seen in previous chapters, it is UNAIDS that has generated the guidelines on bioethics for RCTs and has sought to involve those directly affected by RCTs in a consultative process to address on-going as well as newly arising issues. It is also active in addressing questions provoked by the prospect of the implementation of PrEP. Even so brief an outline as this should further underline the complex relations amongst the agencies involved in the HIV field.[3] When local government bodies, companies, collectives and so on are also taken into account, the picture becomes vertiginous. It is a picture that is also topological insofar as these various actors in the shifting HIV assemblage do not simply co-exist but can profoundly affect one another, becoming-with in the specificity of particular eventuations of HIV and PrEP RCTs. In this chapter, we shall trace one such possible co-emergence in relation to PrEP and the AIDS Clock, though to be sure, we will only be able to explore a few of the generative exchanges and relations between them. For instance, while RCTs are assessed for their ethicality, this is mainly restricted to the specific relations between researchers' intentions and the potential effects of the trial on their research subjects. As we have documented above, the surveillance data gathered on rates of infection embody rather static and thus morally and politically loaded epidemiological categories. These, we have argued, presuppose a particular ethical rationale for the trials that is not subject to the same sort of review (despite recognition that the epidemic is changing, see below). Topologically and, perhaps, provocatively we might suggest that the data on which the AIDS Clock draws simultaneously, albeit diffusely and circuitously, supports the same sort of problematic ethicality. To return to the UNFPA mission statement, the emphasis on very specific forms of data that comprise distinct units of measure (in reference to HIV, this distinctiveness takes the form of recorded infections, deaths reported from AIDS, and numbers of people being administered antiretroviral treatments) at once illustrates and enacts a Euclidean model of space/time. The AIDS Clock is, itself, as we go on to describe, a technology that both embodies and performs this model.

Taking the form of a large digital banner readout at the top of the page, the AIDS Clock displays a large number – at the moment of writing this was 39,407,098 and rising. Immediately to the left of this figure, scroll three consecutive texts: 'Every 16 seconds, another person dies of AIDS' followed by 'Every 12 seconds another person contracts HIV' and finally 'That leaves:'. The readout moves upwards by one every 20 or so seconds. To the right of the increasing large number is the text: 'People living with HIV'.

Underneath the banner is what looks like a Mercator projection of a world map that is divided into countries. Moving the cursor over the map brings up the name of the country and a number. At the top right hand corner of the map is a small panel. This is divided into three sections: the uppermost contains the text: 'RESIZE THE MAP'; the middle says: 'All countries resize relative to number of people with HIV'; the bottom reads 'Play'. On pressing 'Play' the map transforms from the usual representation of national borders based on a version of land area into a depiction in which area reflects HIV prevalence. Accompanying this is a short text with an arrow pointing at the now enlarged sections of Sub-Saharan Africa: 'The area of a country now represents the number of people living with HIV'. By moving the cursor over each country, that country's name appears along with a figure representing the presumably estimated number of people with HIV. The countries and figures, which stand out, include South Africa (5.7 million), India (2.5 million) and Nigeria (2.6 million).

Here we have, then, a seemingly 'objective' depiction of the HIV epidemic as it is distributed across different parts of the world. However, these numbers for national levels of infection do not seem to be directly reflected in the areas of the resized national territories. For instance, India and South Africa take up roughly the same area whereas South Africa should be somewhat larger, and if one were to take into account relative population size, South Africa would be very considerably larger. It should be obvious that we are not appealing for greater 'accuracy' in the map: rather, we are interested in what such a depiction accomplishes. To illustrate, for all the re-scaling, South Africa appears particularly conspicuous, not least because of its prominent – central – position on the map.

On pressing 'Play' there also appears, directly beneath the first panel, a second panel headed 'MENU'. This has three sections named respectively 'Regional Info', 'Relative to Population' and 'About HIV/AIDS'. Clicking on the first two of these yields more information. Regional Info projects a series of pink disks onto regions of the map: moving the cursor over these brings up a panel for that region (for example, 'Sub-Saharan Africa', 'Asia', 'North America and Europe', 'Eastern Europe and Central Asia', 'Oceania') which relates information about the overall number of people with HIV, women (15+), newly infected and AIDS related deaths. Clicking on the disks brings up another panel containing more information about the region. For instance, for 'Sub-Saharan Africa' we are told that this is the region 'most heavily affected by HIV worldwide, accounting for two thirds (67 per cent) of all people living with HIV and for three quarters (75 per cent) of AIDS deaths in 2007...Sub-Saharan Africa's epidemics vary significantly from country to country – with most appearing to have stabilized, although often at very high levels.' However, we are not told what the logic behind this regionalization is (why a categorization between 'North America and Europe' and 'Eastern Europe and Central Asia' that divides Europe? Why 'Sub-Saharan Africa' where there is such wide variation in the incidence of HIV infection across component countries?). Clicking on 'Relative to Population' displays a colour key for the percentage of adults (0–49 years) that are infected with HIV and the reconfigured map is coloured in accordingly (the darkest red designates greater than 20.1 per cent of the population, the lightest pink designates under 1 per cent).

Clicking the final panel of 'MENU' prompts a drop-down menu with the following list of panels: 'Intensifying Prevention', 'Women and Girls', 'Young People', 'Vulnerable Groups' and 'Condom Programming'. Clicking on any of these brings up a text panel that addresses such relevant issues as the differential HIV infection rates between men and women, or between older and younger people, the reasons behind the focus on vulnerable groups or the investment in programmes promoting the use of condom. At the bottom of all but one of these panels is a link which opens up a new UNFPA window which is headed 'Preventing HIV/AIDS': this expands on the topic and provides a series of further links.

Just beneath the map is a thin beige strip at the right of which is the text 'About this map' which links to basic information about the sources of the map. Scrolling down to the bottom of the AIDS Clock webpage there is a large section that links to additional resources. On the left of this, there is slide show entitled 'The Global Epidemic: Fast Facts (click image to zoom)'. Clicking the backwards and forwards tabs takes the reader through a series of 11 slides. For instance, one slide depicts the 'Estimated number of children (>15 years) newly infected with HIV, 2007'. This includes another global map (with named – slightly different – regions) and the regional number and range of child infections. Beneath the map is the overall figure. Another slide comprises a table headed 'Regional HIV and AIDS statistics and features, 2007'. To the right of this bottom section is a list of links to the 2008 Report on global AIDS epidemic, a Media Kit, Multimedia, and a Download of Fast Fact Powerpoint slides. At the very bottom of the AIDS Clock page there are some final links most immediately relevant of which is that named 'About the AIDS Clock'.

Following this link takes us to a page which relays some of the history of the AIDS Clock. Thus we learn that the AIDS Clock was originally launched in 1997 at the United Nations in New York. It was created by UNFPA 'as way to acknowledge both the toll of the epidemic and the partnership that was formed to tackle it'. Moreover, it was a means to allowing people to 'comprehend, in a visual and visceral way, the scale of the epidemic'. The clock as an exhibition went on tour (for example, Toronto, The Hague) before becoming in 2000 a 'web-based feature (that was) improved in 2006 and 2008'. As an advocacy tool the clock's continued functioning 'serves as a reminder that time is running out in many lives and that accelerated measures are needed to reverse the spread of HIV/AIDS'. It is a resource that 'organizations, schools and networks are encouraged to link to and use...in any way they can to spread awareness of the epidemic and the programmes that are combatting it'.

The rationale behind the AIDS Clock is further explicated in a 2006 press release announcing the relaunch of the clock. Accordingly, 'The AIDS Clock reminds us of how pressing our work is', said UNFPA Executive Director Thoraya Ahmed Obaid: 'The clock ticks louder as the number of people living with HIV increases. Behind each number is a face, a family and a circle of loved ones who are also affected. Our goal is to slow down, and eventually turn back the AIDS Clock. Preventing HIV is the key.' The clock and the website thus serve as 'a multimedia advocacy tool' that 'links to regional figures, fact sheets and epidemiology trends, based on information provided by UNAIDS. It also provides links, amongst others, to some of the major campaigns that work to spread awareness of the issue and mobilize effective responses' (UNFPA, 2012).

We have gone into some considerable detail over the AIDS Clock in order to unpack the dual aspects of the Clock, that is, the juxtaposition of two elements in its eventuation. On the one hand, as we have noted, by following the various links from the AIDS Clock website, underpinning the headline figure of 'people living with HIV' and the resizing map are complex arrays of data on different regions, groups, age-ranges and so on. On the other hand, this complexity is distilled – indeed condensed – into a single emotive figure and a dramatically morphing map that is enacted as having global reach and universal affective potency. Our simple point is that the AIDS Clock is a globalizing mechanism that pulls together a range of biomedical data sources that provide the epistemic grounding for a viscerally powerful representation. Both the epistemic (data, the links to scientific reports) and the affective (the headline figures, the morphing map) are presented as accessible, forceful and effective anywhere anytime. These epistemic and affective elements of the AIDS Clock – we might loosely attach them to respectively the enunciatory and the machinic dimensions of the Clock's assemblage – are seen to operate globally because they apparently embody external, universally recognizable parameters or standards. The epistemic embodies the standards of biomedical science or epidemiology; the figure and the morphing map embody the more tacit standards of affect – or what from a constructionist perspective might be called common emotion conventions (which set out the warrant for emotion performances within given social situations, see, for example, Thoits, 1989; Harré, 1986). In other words, the AIDS Clock works globally to assemble its users by operationalizing external pre-given epistemic and affective parameters, standards or conventions. Yet, as we shall argue below, there are good reasons to be circumspect about the AIDS Clock's globalizing credentials. Although intended to raise support, and particularly international donor support for addressing the challenges of the epidemic (most notably what is usually characterized as a 'north/south' asymmetry) it has a curious yet unexplicated relationship to the problematic way in which 'offshore RCTs' take place and, hence, to the particular emergence of PrEP.

RCTs and their ethics, again

As noted repeatedly, randomized control trials as the gold standard of biomedical research into the efficacy of drugs and, in the present case, prophylactics for HIV (PrEP), are generally assumed to apply any time any place. They have universal applicability. However, as we have also

seen throughout the present volume, the concrete testing of PrEP's efficacy and effectiveness is hugely complex. The immense range of what
might be deemed corporeal, social, behavioural, ethical, political and so
on, relations that go into eventuating a PrEP trial have allowed us to trace
the multifarious status of 'gold standard-ness' (see Chapters 4 and 5).
We have also noted how RCTs' accompanying ethical codes of practice,
while on the whole regarded as applicable in all cases, are nevertheless
also held to be problematic (see Chapter 2). Below a trialist explains,
in reference to a controversial trial called ACTG 076 (discussed in some
detail in Chapter 2), how the value of a trial depends on the context
in which it is carried out. Testing a biomedical intervention that is not
known as effective against another that has been demonstrated to be
effective will be regarded as futile in the United States and Europe but,
according to this particular trialist, in Asian or sub-Saharan African countries it may have value:

> If you're taking the point of view of the woman in Thailand [compared
> to a women in the United States or Western Europe], it's probably
> better to be in a placebo-controlled trial, in the long run [even if the
> candidate is not likely to be as effective as an already tested one but
> which is not available in Thailand]... it's better having a 50 percent
> per cent chance of getting the drug [through randomization]. If you're
> testing two active regimens against each other, there's a 100 percent
> chance of getting a drug, so you might think that it's better to do it
> that way, from an ethical standpoint. But it really depends on where
> you are, what you're looking at. (Trialist – R22)

It is worth reiterating a quote from the same respondent used in
Chapter 4, not least because it forcefully underlines the point that there
is a tension between the globalizing and the localizing aspects of the
PrEP trials.

> And, in fact, it's not really consistent with the current Helsinki
> Guidelines [that] you should test against a known treatment. On the
> other hand, one African said at a meeting that I attended in Europe – a
> European body that was discussing this – it's not really of any value to
> us to show that it's not as good as what's used in the US, because that
> means...once you show that, then it won't be used at all. Whereas
> if you show that a possibly inferior regimen, but much more prac-
> tical, works against the placebo, then it will be used, and there will be
> benefit. (Trialist R22)

In reference to our discussion of topology, what is especially pertinent about these statements is how the international HIV field simultaneously does *and* does not recognize how difference emerges across the epidemic and the RCTs that are designed to combat it.

At base, there is a complex interplay between the singularity and diversity, between the difference and similarity, entailed in RCTs and their attendant bioethics. As noted repeatedly, similarity and singularity are mediated through common 'calibrating technologies' such as the RCT, bioethics and, as we have seen, the AIDS Clock. A Euclidian space has been generated by these technologies in which different events (RCTs, efficacy, ethics, infections) can be situated, measured, compared and aggregated. At the same time there is difference being enacted. We see this in the above quotes which point to the contingencies of what is ethical or epistemically robust – placebo-using trials can be ethically appropriate to local circumstances.[4] Similarly, through use of the device of the AIDS Clock all the (partial) differences depicted in the map are abstracted and fed into a single clock figure that, as with the original clock, aims to allow people 'to comprehend, in a visual and visceral way, the scale of the epidemic'.[5] Yet, to repeat, the website as a whole includes multiple means of invoking regional, national and demographic differences in the epidemic.

There are a number of interconnected issues to develop from the foregoing discussions of these 'topological tensions' at the heart of the AIDS Clock and the RCTs and their bioethics. By way of setting the scene, we can note that within what seems like a Euclidean space where external 'global' parameters describe the connections between points, we find that connections develop between disparate points. Crucially, the grounds or principles underpinning these connections are themselves emergent. The irony is that such grounds or principles can in their turn be seemingly generative of a quasi-Euclidian space. In other words, emergent principles of connection can give rise, ostensibly, to external, quasi-Euclidean, criteria (say epistemic or ethical). However, as we have been at pains to note throughout the book, these are complexly related to any particular eventuation. As we saw with regard to 'gold standard-ness', such criteria are simultaneously instantiated and emergent in particular events, but also serve as both a prospect or attractor and its (imprecise) opposite, namely, an anti-attractor that 'precipitates' counter-prospects.

Topological trajectories I: PrEP as medium...

Firstly, in exploring the complexities of these assemblages, we need to be sensitive to the ways in which divergent eventuations of the local can topologically connect. In the above quotes from Trialist 22, we see how the local in the form of the situated utility of placebo-using RCTs also evokes a nexus or assemblage of locals: different RCT sites are united not by their adherence to an external epistemic (epidemiological) framework or on the basis of a standard ethical considerations (Helsinki Guidelines) but through emergent, local contingencies and practicalities associated with the situated utility of placebo-using RCTs. There is a bringing together – a reterritorialization – of divergent points in the HIV assemblage according to emergent, common 'criteria'. We see a parallel evocation of this emergent connectivity in the morphing of the AIDS Clock map described above. Reminiscent of topological deformation, new relations emerge with this morphing: the re-sizing of various countries brings into focus new types of proximity, not based on cartography, but on new classifications in terms of, for instance, the difference between initial and subsequent area size, or the rate of re-sizing (where size denotes levels of HIV infection). The point here is that emergent criteria of similarity are eventuated that draw together otherwise distal entities or points (for example, countries).

Here is another example of this emergent topological connectivity. As before, we can note initially the way in which the numbers, and the process of calculation, do and do not matter. In an article by Page-Shafer et al. (2005), there is a statement to the effect that the early PrEP trial in Cambodia was proposed for female sex workers because HIV incidence and prevalence was amongst the highest in the Asia-Pacific region. They further qualify the decision to use Cambodian female sex workers by noting that although Tenofovir (TDF) was being tested in Africa, 'the results of these investigations might not be directly relevant to women in Asia, because of differences in overall health status, body size, attitudes to medical intervention, and possibly genetic factors' (2005:1499). Here we see how difference is articulated according to a Euclidean logic. The bodies in Asia and Africa are enacted as different but ultimately they can be treated as comparable through the deployment of the appropriate pharmaceutical compound. Yet, at the same time there is some consideration of the complex social relations that may give shape to this apparently distinct and stable technical space of biomedical intervention. We see this when the authors address how what can count as a 'viable' research population is affected by other factors:

> We also perceived that the constraint on US funded agencies with respect to sex-worker-related-projects [this refers to PEPFAR President's Emergency Plan for AIDS relief] might have contributed

to a sense of disenfranchisement among some groups. (Page-Shafer et al., 2005:1500)

As we have noted, PEPFAR funding at the time included 'the anti-prostitution loyalty oath' which required organizations to state that they were opposed to prostitution and sex trafficking, and were thus prohibited from continuing support to sex workers.[6] With what is taken to be the benefit of hindsight, Page-Shafer et al. (2005) are able to claim that the political context caused hostility toward the trial. The latter was, in their view mistakenly, linked to the US's moralistic outlawing of safe sex programmes, programmes regarded by those working to protect sex workers from HIV infection as an occupational hazard. That is, a risk incurred by the work practice which needed to be addressed through programmes of support. However, what Page-Shafer et al. (2005) do not recognize is that there was and, indeed, continues to be a worrisome link between 'donor' countries with the funds to carry out trials, the production of globalized figures for HIV infection and so on, and what does or doesn't take place at the local level.

At the risk of introducing what may be an overly constricted account, it can be recognized that there is a relationship between such international funding policies as PEPFAR[7] and attitudes to trials undertaken by researchers who are based in the countries of origin of such international funding initiatives. That is to say, potential trial participants can be suspicious of those who promote and conduct trials – trials that are seen to be selective and do not address the exigencies of populations at risk of HIV infection (such as sex workers). However, as we have discussed in Chapter 2, opposition to such trials was articulated almost exclusively in terms of their unsatisfactory bioethics. Here, we suggest that alongside such ethics-grounded responses, local scepticism also draws on a range of other factors. For instance, a long history of western colonization, on-going sex tourism involving men from donor or trial-sponsoring countries, and the mediated contrasts between the local extremes of poverty and the affluent conditions of donor countries will also arguably contribute to doubts about biomedical researchers' motives for setting up clinical trials in a country such as Cambodia or Cameroon.

In sum, the application of a morally-directed aid program in PEPFAR generates not only the perception of local disenfranchisement, but also a political reaction that, drawing on a sense of past colonial exploits, opens up the possibility for new connections amongst potential trial populations such as sex workers or drug users. In this respect, one pertinent example is that of the Network of Sex Work Projects which brought together sex workers from a number of countries including Bangladesh, Brazil, Cambodia, Mali and Thailand to produce a 13-minute documentary called 'Taking the Pledge'. The documentary comprises different individuals discussing how the 'anti-prostitution pledge' – a condition for receiving USAID and PEPFAR funds – deleteriously affected the living conditions of sex workers and corroded effective prevention programmes (Network of Sex Work Projects, 2006).

In reviewing the early PrEP RCTs and the controversies that arose around them, we see how the application of external moral and technical parameters has the unintended consequence of facilitating the emergence of topological connections across sex worker groups. These parameters affectively serve as anti-attractors that facilitate the emergence – the reterritorialization – of a new assemblage.

In some respects, these local cultural sentiments toward HIV can be partly attributed to the shifting allegiances and changing programmes (in which PrEP is caught up) amongst various actors within US HIV science field (which include advocacy groups, researchers, government institutions and pharmaceutical companies). As Robert Grant, Principal Investigator for iPrEX RCT recounted in a detailed email in 2008 in which he described the context in which he sought to establish the RCT:

> ...Oddly, I think any prevention in MSM (men who have sex with men), except 'behavioral' interventions is also orphaned. The NIH HIV Prevention Trials Network has some openly gay men.... but the network always ends up doing studies in African women. Even to this day, the CHAMP (The Community HIV/AIDS Mobilisation Project) focus is explicitly on 'Domestic' prevention, and not on prevention in MSM.... how much this 'Domestic' focus is really (the) politically acceptable face for an MSM agenda – it is not clear to me.
>
> How did MSM get left out of the prevention agenda? I think it is because of the theory of 'risk compensation' – MSM are thought to be fully empowered actors who should protect themselves. In contrast, women, female sex workers, IDU are victims who need assistance.
>
> I believe our PrEP trial in MSM was funded, by the way, not because we convinced anyone that MSM had a right to know if PrEP worked for them. Rather, at the time, it seemed that we had capacity to do high quality PrEP research in MSM while all other PrEP trials were failing.

In this example we see a connection across prevention RCT initiatives being made: what ties these together is MSM, or rather their exclusion as a trial population because they were seen to be 'fully empowered'. To qualify they had to, our respondent suggests, perhaps come under the guise of a broader category of 'the domestic'. More crucially, this moral judgement of MSM comes to be laid aside when failures elsewhere in other trials render them a viable experimental population. The point again is that rather than external parameters that determine what groups possess eligibility for PrEP trials, these parameters are subverted, or else they precipitate emergent forms of qualification. In bringing MSM into the same category as African women (in linking them all together as appropriate PrEP trial participants) new contingent criteria are mobilized. In topological terms, we might say there is a shift from a more constricted set of parameters (for example, homeomorphic) to a more permissive set in which MSM become aligned with African women (for example, homotopic). Put another way, what this and previous examples illustrate is the emergence of novel spatializations – a de- and re-territorialization of a part of the HIV assemblage.

While this discussion has focused on the enactment of new experimental subjects – that is, the identification and re-valuation of a previously marginal trial population – through PrEP, we should not forget that should PrEP become more generally available (as has recently taken place with FDA approval in the US for prescribing Truvada as a pre-exposure prophylaxis) a new set of topological shifts are likely to take place and new patterns of identification and differentiation, of connection and disconnection, instituted. At minimum, we might expect that with PrEP's availability will come the need for new HIV antibody testing services, new health monitoring for possible drug side-effects, and new ways of conceptualizing risk and prevention. But so, too, may emerge new sexual subjects as practices alter along with changed risk of infection. Those previously using a condom to protect themselves might find PrEP a suitable alternative or a form of extra protection. In other words, PrEP is more than likely to contribute both to the heterogeneity of the epidemic that has been observed with the introduction of antiretroviral treatments (Flowers, 2001; Race, 2001; Rosengarten, 2009) and to new connectivities as different groups find unexpected common cause.

Topological trajectories II: PrEP as product...

So PrEP can serve as a 'parameter' through which bodies are rendered comparable (not least through the conduct of RCTs), but crucially it is also a generator of difference which can, in a topological involution, render novel comparabilities or connections. In other words, PrEP serves as a medium through which similarities and differences, connections and disconnections, are played out. However, PrEP is also a product – an actual entity – within an assemblage from which it emerges through a parallel process of identification and differentiation, connection and disconnection. At the most obvious level, the design of the PrEP trials is identified with and differentiated from other RCTs for biomedical prevention or treatment technologies.

One of our respondents emailed the following:

> In contrast, in 2004, advocacy groups with any interest in HIV prevention were quite disconnected from each other:
>
> There were organizations advocating for vaccines, including AVAC, which was closely aligned with NIH [National Institutes of Health], HVTN [HIV Vaccines Trials Network], IAVI [International AIDS Vaccine Initiative], and vaccine manufacturers. Although AVAC helped PREP in important ways, they were criticized for supporting a competing concept. This may have limited their advocacy.
>
> There were also organizations advocating for topical microbicides, in close alignment with a feminist movement. Interestingly, topical microbicide advocates were often the most hostile to PREP. The Nigeria PREP trial site, for example, closed partly because the site investigator was focused on public debates driven by the topical microbicide advocates.... (R15)

From this it would appear that PrEP itself was marginalized in various ways: set into a different category of intervention. A parallel narrative of categorical differentiation was set out by another of our respondents in the following way:

> There are a lot of the same issues with PrEP trials as with vaccine and topical microbicide trials but one of the weird things about PrEP was that at the same time that Act Up Paris was protesting vigorously, two huge microbicide efficacy trials were getting underway, sponsored by NIH, both in Africa, neither with any guarantee of treatment to women who became infected. You know, basically ... probably 90 per cent of the things that Act Up Paris were complaining about in the PrEP trials, which were equally applicable to these microbicide trials, nobody was saying a word. I can only speculate, obviously, but the impression that I came away with was that it was because a drug that was involved. Because they [vaccines and topical microbicides] weren't somehow in that same box, they were being ignored. And that's kind of frustrating! (R24)

The reference to 'frustrating' is a comment on the ethics of the trials: Act UP Paris disputed the particular ethics of PrEP RCTs to the neglect of what the respondent saw as very similar, if not identical, ethical issues, raised by the vaccine and topical microbicide trials. There is, in this respondent's view, an illegitimate differentiation being enacted whereby PrEP, in this moment, emerges as an 'other' to topical microbicides on the basis of its RCT's supposed ethical shortcomings – shortcomings which the respondent does not accept insofar as they are of more general applicability. Instead R24 posits a different 'real' reason – namely that PrEP involves 'drugs' whereas microbicides do not.

R24 does not elaborate on why the fact that PrEP entails the administering of drugs should yield a hostile response, and R15 only hints at the reasons behind the resistance to PrEP by feminist and other supporters of topical microbicides. Nevertheless, we can point to the way in which – in the early stages of PrEP's eventuation – what it 'was' was deeply affected by its differentiation from other initiatives. On this score, it was initially marginal within the HIV assemblage.

Topological trajectories III: PrEP as affect...

So far, we have sketched how PrEP is entangled in, and emergent from, a number of patterns of identification and differentiation that marks a particular topology of the HIV assemblage. It will be obvious that our account of the composition of this assemblage entails a relatively limited array of elements: African women, MSM, microbicides, various actors involved in the design, funding, implementation or cessation of RCTs. Our account is limited in part because we have attended mainly to the 'enunciatory' elements of this assemblage to the neglect the 'machinic'. Nevertheless, in the enunciatory patterns we have considered above (for example, the play of epistemic and ethical categorizations), we have also glimpsed the machinic, specifically in the evocation of affect. The comments of several of our respondents suggest that to work with PrEP is to be moved by a range of affects and to experience a panoply of emotions. If we were to abstract these affects and emotions through our engagement with the field of PrEP, we could mention frustration, aggravation, commitment, resilience, perseverance, anger, competitiveness, rigour, pity, and, on occasion, joy.

Now, one of the advantages of the topological perspective being enacted here is that it affords a sensibility toward identifications or connections that might otherwise be considered odd or uncommon or eccentric or occluded. We have already remarked on how the AIDS

Clock aims to enable apprehension 'in a visual and visceral way, the scale of the epidemic'. Similarly, the 'gold standard-ly' principles that are associated with RCTs and their bioethics are affective insofar as they provoke a potent sense of what is the correct way of intervening in the epidemic. Of course, all this is further complicated by the contingences that we have attempted to follow: the local implementation of RCTs yields, as noted immediately above, by a spectrum of other affects. The key point we wish to draw out is that this affective dimension also allows us to trace, necessarily speculatively given that affects are not readily accessible (see below), the substantive topologies that connect different eventuations of and within the HIV assemblage – in particular, those between the AIDS Clock and PrEP trials.

However, in order to do this, we need first to clarify what we mean by affect. Here, affect is treated as a broader category than emotion. It is concerned with the impact on bodies given their corporeal, perceptual and reactive capacities. As such affect is a part of the machinic aspect of assemblages (see Deleuze and Guattari, 1988; also Massumi, 2002, and Bennett, 2010). The amorphousness of affect (when it becomes emotion it has been mediated by emotion conventions – Michael, 2011) means that affects can draw links between apparently disparate events. To be affected by one event means that one might be predisposed to be affected by, or respond to, an altogether seemingly different event. However, this amorphousness does mean that affect is not easy to grasp empirically: in the end, an element of extrapolation, indeed, of speculation, seems to be unavoidable.

In the present case, we can suggest that the affects generated by the event of the AIDS Clock can have implications in relation to the eventuation of PrEP RCTs and their bioethics, and vice versa. In other words, the relation between the AIDS Clock and PrEP can be de- and re-territorialized in topologically interesting and, as we shall see, differential, ways.

As we have noted above, the symbol that is the AIDS Clock is designed to have an affective impact, to act as a motivational spur to combat the steady increase in infections. Yet its readership remains undifferentiated – anyone anywhere, it seems, will be responsive to its affects. Over and above literacy let alone digital divides, the data displayed in the AIDS Clock is most likely to affect western actors, not least those who are directly implicated in decisions that affect the epidemic such as, most relevantly in the present discussion, the scientists and ethicists engaged in designing and conducting PREP RCTs. To reiterate, the clinical trialling of PrEP is technically best conducted at sites of relatively elevated HIV incidence where prevention is comparatively poor such that the effects of PrEP can be detected clinically as useful data. Under such circumstances, the presence of the trial may not only reduce the incidence of infection (through the ethically standardized prevention counselling) but also increase the risk of infection through the unintended consequence of PrEP coming to be seen as a replacement for condom use. In essence, PrEP RCTs can locally generate infections that eventually end up adding to the generic figure of HIV infections that are cumulatively marked by the AIDS Clock. The affective topology is that the surveillance data displayed in the Clock works back to motivate those very scientists.

To be sure, it is a speculative topological trajectory that we have outlined here. The aim has not been to show definitively how affects have shaped the particular eventuation of trials – to operationalize such a project would be empirically controversial to say the least: how does one trace unmediated affects when what we 'see' or depict academically is always already mediated (especially by emotion conventions)? Other modes of engagement are needed – not least 'non representational' ones (see, for example, Thrift, 2008). Be that as it may, our objective here has been to use the motif of affect as a suggestive means of exploring possible topological connections between otherwise distal points in the HIV assemblage. We shall return to a further implication of this strategy below.

To summarize this section, we have attempted to unravel a few of the many complexities of PrEP RCTs through the use of topological thinking. In particular, we have tried to identify a few of those rhizomic moments where disparate parts of the HIV assemblage have come together, or even where the rhizomic and rootish, the emergent and the standardized, or the topological and the Euclidian themselves – have folded into each other. We are fully aware that we have barely scratched the (folded) surface of these complex relationalities but we do hope that the preceding has gone some little distance to illustrating, if not wholly illuminating, the possibilities offered by topological thinking in such an empirical field.

Conclusion: Topologizing our topology ...

It will not have escaped notice in the preceding account that we have, ourselves, attempted to avoid globalizing and Euclidean tendencies. While we have argued that new general criteria or parameters emerge, the view that such a process of emergence is local and contingent can itself be globalized, that is, rendered an external parameter. In other words, emergence and contingency become raised to abstracted principles no less universalizing than those embodied in the 'gold standard' of RCTs – local contingency, and indeed topology, apply anytime anywhere. Elsewhere (Michael and Rosengarten, 2012b), we have elaborated this point, suggesting that what may be of continuing importance is to interrogate the topological relations between the disciplines of topology and social science. However, in the present case, we will follow another topological twist. In what follows, we will connect our own faltering attempts at a topological social science to an example of poetry and its literary analysis that challenges the ways in which Euclidean conceptions of time, space and the individual continue to shape intervention in the HIV epidemic.

However, before that, we should just note that some of the notions – 'HIV positive' and 'epidemic' – that we ourselves have used more or less unproblematically throughout this book (to draw together different trial events, for instance) can benefit from topological analysis. So far we have drawn on a topological sensibility to trace how distant entities and events might be closer together than is at first apparent. However, topology also allows us to explore how what seem to lie close together – to be identical, even – are situated at considerable distances from one another, or belong to rather different categories.

As may be evident from our earlier description, the UNAIDS Clock generates a sense of urgency about infection rates (numbers). It also contributes to a style of quantification with worrisome political effects. The process of quantification depends on an epidemic that is modelled according to the bifurcation of 'global/local' 'north/south' as well as a series of other assumed differences. Over the past thirty years or so, the grounds for the 'global/local' or 'north/south' have not much shifted, nor have there been substantial changes in the assumed differences that underpin the usual epidemiological categories (categories typically insensitive to heterogeneous dynamics of cultures). Perhaps the most instructive example of this is the continued reliance on a distinction between 'HIV positive' and 'HIV negative' status rather than differences within the category of 'HIV positive' and within different self-perceptions of 'HIV negative' status (see Flowers, 2001; Rosengarten, 2009). We refer here to important studies that show that those who have HIV positive status but whose virus is suppressed by anti-retroviral drugs are very unlikely to be able to transmit the virus (Cohen et al., 2011). Other studies suggest that those who act (knowingly or unknowingly) as if HIV negative, but are in an acute stage of infection (which involves greater amounts of viral particles in bodily fluids such as semen, vaginal secretions and blood), are likely to pose a risk of transmission (Saxton et al., 2012; van Sighem et al., 2012). Here, then, we see, that the seemingly external parameters of 'HIV positive' and ' HIV negative' have, with the benefit of hindsight, been doing 'topological work', drawing disparate groups together under single categories.

This insight also has implications for another basic concept within the HIV field, namely that of 'epidemic'. Rather than a global epidemic that draws together all HIV infection, it has become possible to address 'concentrated epidemics'; that is, based on tracing high rates of infections amongst, for instance, MSM, discrete epidemics of HIV infection that lie 'within', or in place of, 'generalised epidemics' can be identified. Epidemics traced through heterosexual transmission are not unproblematically comparable with epidemics traced through MSM anal intercourse: that is to say, these instantiations of HIV transmission are not comfortably ascribable to a singular 'global epidemic'.

The overarching point is that both the parameters of 'HIV positive' and 'epidemic' are themselves topologically emergent. Part of the ethos of topology is, therefore, to reflect on the ways that categories, parameters and concepts and their operations – which mediate a topological analysis – would themselves be illuminated through a topological analysis.

Pushing this spirit of topologizing our own topology a little further, we can develop some connections with a rather different analytic field (thus topologizing our social scientific perspective on the HIV filed, and, indeed, topology). To this end we draw on a commentary by the literary theorist Neville Hoad (2010) of the well-known South African HIV prevention campaign 'Love Life'.[8] Although Hoad's analysis of the epidemic that informs his critique of 'Love Life' does not quite echo the sort of conceptual approach we have followed in this volume, his commentary is no less a poignant account of the political, ethical and, indeed, medical stakes in difference. He notes how the 'Love Life' campaign of mainly billboard advertising – though it also entailed the promotion of T-shirts with the logo 'HIV positive' – was insistent on breaking the silence around HIV. Despite the well-meaning intentions behind it and endorsements from the likes of Nelson Mandela and others, it nevertheless enacted a public and, crucially, a universalized experience of pain and trauma, and embodied a presumption that this one strategy could apply for all those people who were 'HIV positive'. As a counter to this, Hoad draws on a poem by Phaswane Mpe, and includes in his citing of it the following line: 'silence too is love', suggesting it tells us of more intimate and complex sets of experiences of living with HIV/AIDS. In his words:

That the poem itself breaks a silence while insisting 'silence too is love', marks a paradox that must invoke an idea of publicness, not just as collective empowerment, but also as the site of shame, stigma, and exposure, that there might be something unspeakable about both suffering and love. (Hoad, 2010:141)

Later, in the same essay, Hoad goes on to critique the use of numbers:

Numbers as indices of aggregates and averages cannot account for differential experiences within their mode of representation. An HIV diagnosis means very different things in terms of the geographical location, class, race, and gender designation of the person receiving that diagnosis in terms of treatment options, social support, employment, and immigration options, and so on... On the other hand, by leaving so much to the imagination, numbers might be deeply ethical and potentially democratic, though any imagining of a public imagination must brace itself for categories like prejudice, xenophobia and stigma. When I hear a number, my first thought is 'pick one', but I know there are professions in which being responsible to, with and for numbers is important. I also know that hidden in those figures are deep and on going histories of governmentality and sovereignty, stories of emergent and now hegemonic sciences of demography, epidemiology, the hegemony of the modern state and the glimpses of its shifting role under neoliberalism – I cannot yet say demise. (2010:146)

Despite their intent to address the urgency of rising infections, both the AIDS Clock and the PrEP RCTs restrict the possibilities that numbers might offer. Along with Hoad, we too have been asking, albeit in a different idiom, 'how do they pick their numbers'? Although those numbers enact the HIV field as if it were there well before the design of a clock or a RCT, it is our basic argument that these devices are part of the making of numbers and the field (and, as we hoped to have illustrated in this chapter, they can work off each other in so doing). That is to say, the numbers are not independent of the temporal-spatial way in which the epidemic is laid out in the mapping of the UNAIDS Clock and the conduct of PrEP RCTs. So, again alongside Hoad, we might ask what follows in the wake of the selection of numbers by the Clock and RCTs. What bearing does the intertwining of these devices have on the epidemic? As Hoad suggests, these numbers carry a multitude of histories that frame the epidemic in very particular ways. But because numbers have their specific limitations and productivities, because they leave 'so much to the imagination' they also, as we have noted in relation to the notion of the 'event', open up possibilities – they can serve as anti-attractors that draw the event of HIV and PrEP in new directions that are in Hoad's words 'deeply ethical and potentially democratic'.

In the next, concluding, chapter, we summarize and reflect on the previous chapters. However, we also want to begin to expand on the virtualities entailed in the analytic perspective (with its key concepts of event, assemblage, topology, becoming-with, etc.) developed and applied in the foregoing. Specifically, we will explore a topological twist cum virtuality of our own – one that, on the one hand, re-territorializes our disciplinary situation through a potential collaboration with 'speculative' design and trialists and, on the other, opens out onto the prospect of a re-working of the PrEP RCT so that it becomes a site for inventive problem-making.

7
Conclusion: Eventuating the Methodology of Trials

From project to prospect

This book has been about biomedical innovation and the practical, local, analytic, distributed efforts to determine whether a relatively mundane intervention (a pre-existing pharmaceutical drug or a combination of pre-existing pharmaceutical drugs for the treatment of HIV infections) amounts to a viable prophylactic against HIV infection. Toward the beginning of this book, we drew a contrast between mundane and exotic technologies as a way of situating PrEP and yet, as we have illustrated throughout, this distinction is not easy to sustain (see especially Chapter 3). All sorts of novelties and multiplicities flow in the wake of PrEP's testing – novel bodies, relations, virus, pharmaceuticals, politics, clinical and social arguments. So, despite the comparative lack of innovation that ostensibly marks PrEP, it has occasioned all sorts of inventiveness. In this respect it is no different from other sorts of mundane technology which have precipitated novelty (conversely, it is the mirror image of supposedly exotic technologies which simply reproduce or reinforce existing values or functions – see, for example, Michael, 2000; Barry, 2001). So, this book has concerned itself with tracing some of the patterns of invention and non-invention that have characterized the recent history of PrEP, its randomized control trialling and accompanying bioethics.

Throughout this project, we have attempted to engage with PrEP, PrEP RCTs and bioethics as 'things' – heterogeneous, multiple, complex, emergent, processual – opening out onto virtual prospects. So while we have investigated several of the many ways in which PrEP, RCTs and bioethics are singularized, quantified, 'object-fied' against external parameters or criteria (we have focused on the epistemic and the ethical – see Chapter 4), we have also explored the diverse even-tuations of PrEP, PrEP RCTs and bioethics, and the co-emergence of numerous parameters with which they are enacted and evaluated (see Chapter 5). This has meant that our perspective on innovation has been aligned with those approaches in the literature that can be broadly called 'constructionist' (see Chapter 3). In keeping with these, we have not been overly interested in whether PrEP RCTs have been successful in the endeavour to demonstrate PrEP efficacy or, indeed, whether the advocates and potential users of PrEP have deemed it a viable preven-tion option or not. Rather, our focus has been on the ways in which 'success' or 'viable' are themselves emergent categories – though, of course, 'success' in the present case, as can equally be said of 'viable,' has taken on many guises that range from standard measures of effi-cacy through to the avoidance of police victimization by intravenous drug users. In other words, we have not been interested in 'success' as a distinct disjuncture, or a moment of discrete novelty. Instead, we have attended to the complex co-emergence of various parameters (which might be used to assess 'success' or 'failure' along various lines including – admixtures of – efficacy, politics, ethics, methodology) along with their 'things' (which might incorporate bodies, sexual rela-tions, gendered relations of power, the ethics of offshore trials, the robustness of clinical data, the local institutional status of sex workers or intravenous drug users, and so on and so forth). On this score, we have also treated PrEP as a 'thing' which is also eventuated through more distantiated and topological relations (Chapter 6).

Needless to say, our particular reworking of innovation rests on our version of the event. The event or, better, the event-uation of PrEP, PrEP RCTs and bioethics is heterogeneous, multiple, complex, emergent, processual, opening out onto virtual prospects, as we put it above. This close link between 'things' and 'events' should come as no surprise (not least in light of Whitehead's own use of, respectively, 'actual entities' and 'actual occasions' – see Halewood and Michael, 2008). What some-thing 'is' thus lies in its process of becoming, its eventuation and, as we have seen, this is complex, folded, multiple and prospective.

Now, our specific view of event and eventuation has been shaped by the 'case' of PrEP itself. We have insisted that PrEP has not been a 'mere' illustration of our particular perspective on process-oriented social science. Indeed, we have tried to 'flatten' the relative statuses of theory, method and empirical material. Our engagement with PrEP obliged us to rethink the category of event, not least in relation to abstraction (specifi-cally the abstractions of gold standard-ness – see Chapters 4 and 5).

However, we do have to admit that methodologically we have not exactly been adventurous – we have, in similar fashion to much work in social studies of science, and social science more generally, drawn on a limited array of techniques for gathering data (see Chapter 3). Data have been derived from interviews with trialists, email communications with key actors, observations at conferences, official documentation, news media accounts of various conflicts, institutional websites and so on. Such methods are no less performative than the discourses, accounts, statistics, reportage, rhetorics they gather up. Social scientific methods likewise enact a world in which various elements are 'othered' as John Law might put it (Law, 2004). But further, the event of data gathering (and analysis) is, itself, an eventuation that is open, prospective. We have attempted to signal this openness – or inconclusion – by revisiting the same PrEP RCT events, each time providing a different account. Nevertheless, we might want to consider if there are ways of doing social science work which are methodologically more open to this openness. Indeed, we might ask whether there are ways of doing social and biomedical science *together* – in collaboration – where this openness, these prospective dimensions of (testing and using) PrEP are proactively engaged. In the latter parts of this chapter, we will begin to address the prospects of addressing the prospective by setting out a sketch for a collaboration with speculative design that facilitates 'inventive problem-making'.

But before we do so, we need to revisit our own recounting of PrEP in relation to the history of research into the prevention of HIV. When we embarked on research into this field and, even later, when we began writing this book, it was pretty obvious that PrEP was very much an underdog intervention, an option by and large consigned to the margins of the field. Vaccines and topical microbicides received far more attention from the HIV research community. Indeed PrEP was in some quarters subject to outright hostility amongst HIV prevention advocates and people affected by HIV. Some organizations have opposed its introduction, and the AIDS Healthcare Foundation, in particular, has mounted a provocative campaign against its approval: 'If you love Vioxx you'll love PrEP', read one poster displayed on bus shelters near the White House Washington DC, comparing PrEP to the painkilling drug that was withdrawn in 2004 when it was linked with heart attacks.

But this is a fast shifting field and suddenly – and certainly, for us, unexpectedly – PrEP has risen to prominence even over the course of writing this book. We began by pointing out that PrEP had very recently been approved by the FDA (United States Federal Drug Administration). As we conclude, we find not only has the field shifted but we, too, have moved from observers of the process of PrEP emergence into a more active role that might indeed have an impact on how this should take place. Through our many engagements with the HIV field, we have come to be included in discussions about where and how PrEP might be implemented. However, before elaborating on this 'new' dimension of our own becoming-with, alongside PrEP's own becoming-with, we want to reflect on how it is that we did not foresee such an outcome, that is, PrEP's ontological shift from 'controversial proposal' to 'problematic promise'.

Most importantly, we do not especially see our apparent lack of foresight as a failure of our predictive powers. PrEP is ontologically multiple and some constituent relationalities are inevitably less available to analysis than others. The present eventuation of PrEP as a seemingly viable prophylactic drug is something that is, of course, open to study – how this dramatic change of status came about is a question worth addressing and we will do this in a preliminary way below. Secondly, and more interestingly, the turnaround in PrEP's fortunes simply serves to reinforce the potential value of doing process-oriented research – of engaging with the virtualities onto which a thing such as PrEP opens out. This is simply to underline our previous point: that we need to find methods that can facilitate an engagement with the prospective.

The priority of PrEP

The FDA announcement approving PrEP on 16 July 2012, for prescribing in the US to people tested HIV negative included the following statements on its website:[1]

> As part of PrEP, HIV-uninfected individuals who are at high risk will take Truvada daily to lower their chances of becoming infected with HIV should they be exposed to the virus. A PrEP indication means Truvada is approved for use as part of a comprehensive HIV prevention strategy that includes other prevention methods, such as safe sex practices, risk reduction counseling [sic], and regular HIV testing.
>
> 'Today's approval marks an important milestone in our fight against HIV,' said FDA Commissioner Margaret A. Hamburg, M.D. Every year, about 50,000 U.S. adults and adolescents are diagnosed with HIV infection, despite the availability of prevention methods and strategies to educate, test, and care for people living with the disease. New treatments as well as prevention methods are needed to fight the HIV epidemic in this country.

As a part of this action, the FDA is strengthening Truvada's Boxed Warning to alert health care professionals and uninfected individuals that Truvada for PrEP must only be used by individuals who are confirmed to be HIV-negative prior to prescribing the drug and at least every three months during use. The drug is contraindicated for PrEP in individuals with unknown or positive HIV status. The FDA strongly recommends against such use.

This approval is in some ways quite surprising given the epistemic disarray of the collective data across the trials, as we have documented in this book. Of course, the viability of PrEP is hedged with key provisos, most notably that users need to be HIV negative, which requires regular testing and which, itself, demands a range of commitments and resources. There is, then, an issue around the implementability of PrEP.

This was echoed in another document. Just prior to the 2012 International AIDS Conference in Washington DC, WHO held a two-day meeting inviting those involved in PrEP RCTs and advocacy organizations to develop guidelines for such studies. A small booklet was distributed at this meeting. Its opening included the statement:

> Although the evidence of effectiveness is strong, it remains unclear how PrEP may best be implemented and scaled up in settings where its use might be most beneficial. While the effects on risk behaviours, values, preferences and resource costs have been studied in conjunction with the clinical trials, they are not well understood in actual application, and so the feasibility of PrEP implementation is not known. Therefore, experience with using PrEP outside the context of the controlled clinical trial is needed. (WHO, 2012b:3)

This is a point we have raised many times, namely that the RCTs' exclusionary focus tends to leave effectiveness (and implementation) a relative mystery, or rather collapses them into the concept of efficacy (see, for example, our discussion in Chapter 4). However, this circumspection seemed to be less in evidence in the main Conference (of approximately 23,000 delegates from all over the world). The mood seemed to be one of considerable optimism amongst many of the prominent actors in the field or, at least, this was what was on display. The conference began with a session entitled 'Ending the Epidemic: Turning the Tide Together'.[2] The opening plenary was by Professor Anthony Fauci who happily announced that the use of antiretroviral drugs for prevention – including PrEP but also what is termed 'Treatment as Prevention' or 'TasP' – put on course the possibility that the transmission of HIV may be stopped through various uses of antiretroviral drugs and that new findings bring promise of a possible cure.

This view was presaged by Padian et al. in an article published in 2011. They stated:

> We have entered a new era in HIV prevention whereby priorities have expanded from biomedical discovery to include implementation, effectiveness, and the effect of combination prevention at the population level. However, gaps in knowledge and implementation challenges remain. In this Review we analyse trends in the rapidly changing landscape of HIV prevention, and chart a new path for HIV prevention research that focuses on the implementation of effective and efficient combination prevention strategies to *turn the tide* on the HIV pandemic [our emphasis]. (2011:269)

So, unlike previous conferences that covered numerous disciplines in which oral PrEP attracted little attention, PrEP had now moved centre stage. In part this was made possible by virtue of the results of the iPrEX RCT, the Partners PrEP RCT and a relative newcomer to the stage (although it had been running since 2005), namely, the TDF2 Study in Botswana which contributed to the evidence base on which the FDA's decision to licence Truvada was founded.[3] Indeed just prior to the conference in satellite meetings and during the week-long conference itself, there was much excited discussion about 'demonstration' studies. These studies were either underway or were planned and would be using PrEP 'off label' to establish its effectiveness but also to address nagging questions about how PrEP should be implemented and for whom. In contrast to PrEP RCTs, such studies depart from the inclusion of a placebo arm and are designed on the basis that the intervention is offered to a prescribed number of volunteers form a pre-identified target group (such as MSM) who are willing to be monitored.[4]

If this book opened with mention of this recent FDA approval for PrEP, we have primarily focused on the controversy over early PrEP trials. We have noted that the Cambodian and Cameroon trials were stopped due to initial questions about their ethical status and certain logistical concerns that the subsequent delays posed. We also pointed that the trial conducted by CDC with the Thai health authorities (Ministry of Health, Thailand Bangkok Metropolitan Administration Medical College and Vajira Hospital) continued. In fact, as we have mentioned in the course of our discussions, this trial has been extended a number of times and the results are still pending. The abandonment of trials and the absence of results, when taken together with the complex nexus of findings we have charted, offer at best a dilute and partial hope.

In thinking about the growing enthusiasm for PrEP, and the impact of PrEP's emergence as a serious prophylactic contender on researchers' apprehension of results, we can usefully draw parallels with other cases where scientific 'enthusiasm' has gathered precipitous momentum. For instance, in stem cell research, the Lumelsky protocol for differentiating mouse embryonic stem cells into insulin-producing beta cells was seen as a major breakthrough, leading to a considerable research bandwagon. Yet, it 'should' have been clear from the original results that that there was insulin in the culture medium used to stimulate stem cell differentiation, insulin which was being absorbed then released giving the 'false' impression of beta cell activity (Michael et al., 2007). This sort of collective enthusiasm is not unusual – scientists (and various other invested actors such as funders and charities) become enthused about a particular method or set of results that subsequently come to be judged as problematic. The point is that this should not be regarded as some sort of 'failure' or 'mistake': instead it can be seen as a partial outcome of the 'innovation process' in which, in the context of chronic failure and setback, enthusiastic expectations of success serve to sustain scientists who might otherwise have given up (for example, Borup et al., 2006). This case study simply serves to illustrate the way that seemingly promising results (such as those of TDF2 in Botswana) come to be privileged by a research community in a context of serial failure and/or chronic uncertainty.

Another way of viewing this is that (at the time of writing) the present eventuation of PrEP is oriented-toward and opening-toward an attractor of something like 'a viable prophylactic against HIV infection'. A range of entities including a slogan, data, a conference, the pronouncements of the FDA have come together to eventuate PrEP as a particular sort of thing. However, we would suggest that there is another virtuality here, an anti-attractor in which PrEP's current promising status is broken down, or compromised. Of course, it is possible for us to suggest what form this anti-attractor might take. But we would prefer to take up a different strategy. This entails thinking about how it might be possible methodologically to engage with such virtualities – attractors and anti-attractors alike – in a way that opens up the eventuation of PrEP as an occasion for creatively re-posing the problem, rather than seeing it primarily in terms of a solution, as is currently the case.

Prospecting prophylaxis

If the preceding section presents a version of where 'we are' with PrEP, this final section outlines a version of 'where we might be going' (in both instances, 'we' is placed within inverted commas to connote the fluidity of both the HIV field and our own relation to, and embroilment within, that field). Specifically, we (the authors) want to engage with the virtuality of PrEP (and here PrEP might serve as a proxy for innovation in health technologies more generally).

Let us take a step back first. The book has presented numerous examples of the ways in which RCTs designed to assess the efficacy of PrEP have been met with a variety of issues that trialists either marginalized or struggled to address. Such issues included, minimally, the convolutions of the ethics that were attached by some commentators to the PrEP trials, the varieties of recalcitrance from the trial participants themselves, and the protest actions of a number of activist groups.

Now, these, let us provisionally call them, 'misbehaviours' (Michael, 2012b) can be treated as 'idiotic'. This is not in any way meant as a pejorative term but one which is designed to sensitize us to the limitations of our own thinking. If for the ancient Greeks, the idiot was the person motivated solely by self-interest and thus unwilling to take part in civic political life, for Gilles Deleuze (2004) it was a private thinker who was the arbiter of what was or wasn't knowable (Beckman, 2009). However, later the idiot was transformed into conceptual persona that sought the incomprehensible and the absurd (Deleuze and Guattari, 1994). It is this version that Isabelle Stengers (2005) has championed. Accordingly, the idiot is a 'conceptual character' – a figure that refuses to enter the events in which researchers, for instance, are invested, whose responses make no sense in relation to those events as normally understood (such events can be social as well as biomedical, and the researchers can be social scientists as well as biomedical scientists). As such the idiot can serve to challenge the meaning of such events. Stengers puts it this way:

> the idiot can neither reply nor discuss the issue...(the idiot) does not know...the idiot demands that we slow down, that we don't consider ourselves authorized to believe we possess the meaning of what we know. (Stengers, 2005:995)

Our task turns to how we might grasp the implications of the idiot's nonsensical actions, how:

we bestow efficacy upon the murmurings of the idiot, the 'there is something more important' that is so easy to forget because it 'cannot be taken into account', because the idiot neither objects nor proposes anything that 'counts'. (Stengers, 2005:1001)

In sum, in learning to attend to the nonsensicalness, we become open to a dramatic redefinition of the meaning of the commonsensical event. So, this book has been about this very prospect – redefining what is to count as a randomized control trial, what is to count as the PrEP pill and what is to count as bioethics. Our task has been to 'bestow efficacy upon the murmurings of the idiot' by explicating what, from within the eventuation of the PrEP RCTs (that seek to measure efficacy, that are structured around a very particular version of bioethics), make 'no sense' – what above we, minimally, framed as 'the convolutions of the ethics that were attached by some commentators to the PrEP trials, the varieties of recalcitrance from the participants themselves, and the protest actions of a number of activist groups'.

We can put this another way. John Law (2004) has powerfully reiterated the point that methodology is necessarily performative. Any method (or method assemblage as Law puts it) will entail 'the crafting and enacting of boundaries between presence, manifest absence and Otherness' (2004:85) as certain 'data' are chronically excluded by simply being, within the parameters of the method, un-registerable. Thus 'there will always be Othering' (2004:85). What the idiot, as deployed here, is meant to do is enact this othering in inventive ways which allows us to reconsider 'what we are busy doing'. Of course, such an 'idiotic methodological' process is no less performative – it is involved in the making of the event that is under study (Michael, 2012a). However, the aim is to interject the idiot in order to 'make this making' open, oriented to the virtual and suspicious of the idea that we are in possession of 'the meaning of what we know' and, indeed, what we do.

In the book we have tried to recover some of the 'others' of RCTs and bioethics (by drawing attention to some of the numerous complexities of offshore RCTs) and, albeit tacitly, deployed these idiotically in order to generate a circumspection that we possess the meaning of what we know about, and do within, RCTs and bioethics. However, this has been a reactive process. That is to say, we have sought out some of these others, brought them in from the margins, and argued for a reformulation of the event of RCTs that can accommodate them. In what follows, we want to take this a step further – to use the idiot proactively as a way of variously broadening the parameters of the eventuation of RCTs and bioethics, of rethinking the meaning of data within such an eventuation, and of ensuring that this process is both circumspect and open to the virtual, to the prospective.

If this seems like a tall order for the 'sciences' – social as well as biomedical – then we are fortunate to have a potential, practicable model in the form of Speculative Design. In what follows, we will draw out a number of elements of speculative design that seem to us to be particularly useful in engaging with the virtual in PrEP RCTs and implementation, and of enabling the making of 'inventive problems'. However, given that we will not just be 'doing speculative design' but rather that we will propose an interdisciplinary collaboration across, minimally, speculative design, social science and biomedical science, then we will also need to address how to think such interdisciplinarity in a way that is consonant with our processual perspective.

Unlike mainstream product design, speculative design – which is centrally associated with Bill Gaver and his colleagues at the Interaction Research Studio at Goldsmiths, University of London[5] – is not directly interested in the development of objects that will impact on a pre-specified future (for instance, meet users' known or projected needs). Rather, the prototypes produced by the studio tend to have rather opaque functions. As such they might deploy unusual means to visit on-line information sources and present that information in novel ways. For instance, the 'local barometer' device presented local advertisements taken from a London-based online small ads service but determined by wind speed and direction measured by an anemometer installed on the roof of the user's house. These ads were displayed on beautifully-crafted small screens that could sit on shelves or ledges around the house. It should be clear that the functions of this device are not readily obvious: why use wind speed and direction? The rationale behind the local barometer was to design an object that enabled its user to explore the meanings of their neighbourhood and its environs. One of the unexpected upshots was that the user began to use the advertisements to read wind and weather conditions. This, in turn, begins to raise the possibility of a practical reformulation of the idea of neighbourhood from a social, cultural, economic category to one which included the technical (web connections, electromagnetic networks) and the natural (wind speed, micrometeorology). The local barometer thus serves as an idiot – it does not make sense within the usual eventuation of 'neighbourhood' (or indeed the 'domestic' space). It is open, playful, strange, ambiguous. Practically, it allows for a more interesting re-articulation of the 'problem' – one that can conceptualize 'neighbourhood' through such categories as technonatures or naturecultures (see Michael and Gaver, 2009).

Speculative designers, however, do not derive these devices without first engaging with publics. Such engagements deviate from the standard modes of empirical enquiry in social science, let alone biomedical science or public health. There is no systematic attempt to collect data through tried and tested techniques (interviews, questionnaires, ethnographies, blood tests, etc.), and the material that is gathered is not subjected to the usual processes of analysis which seek out patterns to 'identify' discourses, or grounded theories, or social relations, and so on and so forth. Instead, 'probes' (Boehner et al., 2012) are, paralleling our focus on the virtuality of events, used to address 'what might be'.

Through a mixture of discussion with potential users and consideration of possible issues, likely aesthetics, and possible provocations, probes are designed to allow their users to record idiosyncratic, novel, risky, ambiguous experiences of, for instance, their domestic environment, or their use of energy. Probes can take many forms and are designed afresh for each substantive project. Thus probes may take the form of: a SD card with instructions on how to install this in a camera and a request to take photographs of the boundary of the user's community; an everyday drinking glass with instructions to listen to the sounds in the user's home (by pressing the glass against the walls) and to record those sounds (writing directly onto the glass with the supplied marker pen); or an airmail letter with instructions to write down any confessions about one's energy use. Typically, participants are supplied with a range of probes and it is made clear that they can use and return them as they see fit.

As noted, the role of the probes in the speculative design process is not to 'gather data systematically' that is subject to systematic analysis, but to generate idiosyncratic materials that – 'combined idiosyncratically' with other materials (including policy documents, design histories, magazine articles) – are used to inform the design of the prototype. This process can be fraught in that there is a conscious effort to seek out the odd, the uncomfortable, the unforeseen, the ambiguous, the incomprehensible. In other words, this is a practical attempt to identify the idiotic.

We can perhaps summarize this summary account of speculative design by saying that the idiotic is deployed in order to design the idiotic in order to induce the idiotic. One positive implication is that here are techniques which begin to engage, at several points, with the virtual, and thus open up the opportunity of enabling 'inventive problem-making'. One negative implication is that there is no guarantee that these will work (people can reject probes, or dismiss prototypes – every substantive project is characterized by a renewed and acute sense of the possibility of failure).

How does the work of speculative designers map onto the work presented in this book? We would not want to pre-empt what might be specifically entailed in a collaboration between biomedical scientists, social scientists and speculative designers. However, we can at least sketch some of the parameters to such a collaboration.

As an event of interdisciplinarity we would see such a collaboration in terms of what Barry et al. (2008) call the 'logic of ontology'. This stands in contrast to the 'logic of accountability' where interdisciplinarity is justified in terms of, say, improving interactions between scientists and various non-expert actors (the non-science discipline can stand in as a proxy for the public), or the 'logic of innovation' where, for instance, the non-science discipline identifies potential users of scientific products and as such becomes integral to the innovation cycle. By contrast, the 'logic of ontology' implies that the object of study is transformed by virtue of the fact that, through the interdisciplinary collaborations, it emerges out of both social and natural processes and the relations in-between. For instance, in Born and Barry's (2010) discussion of the PigeonBlog, Beatriz da Costa (a faculty member of the Arts, Computation and Engineering Masters programme at University of California, Irvine) collaborates with scientists measuring air quality. Instead of sensors fixed to static posts set across the city, she attaches GPS-linked sensors to homing pigeons which transmit 'real-time location-based pollution data and imaging to an online mapping and blogging site'.

Born and Barry draw out three implications from the 'public experiment' that is PigeonBlog. First, it involved 'a reconceptualization of air quality as an object of measurement' (2010:114). Secondly, it served in the generation of a 'different kind of public knowledge of air quality: one that highlights the critical significance of its social-geographical variation, and that invites those most affected by this variation to participate in the practices of knowledge production' (2010:114). Thirdly, art is no longer a medium of science communication: rather, it 'draws upon but also augments the resources of science. PigeonBlog makes a scientific contribution, while reconfiguring the objects both of art and of scientific research' (2010:115).

So, within this 'logic of ontology' a number of implications follow for the proposed collaboration between biomedical scientists, social scientists and speculative designers. Perhaps most obviously, through this collaboration a new object of measurement will emerge. This can be translated as new forms of 'data' will become available – data which encompass seemingly heterogeneous elements. Just as the local barometer mediated both the social and the meteorological as 'naturecultures', a prototype might, for instance incorporate ways of simultaneously accessing viral loads and social relations and practices.

Our reluctance to specify, except minimally, these prototypes reflects more than our inexperience in both biomedicine and design. Rather, it signals the fact that these prototypes emerge through initial engagement with participants using probes. In other words, participants are crucial, albeit in an oblique way, in the design process that goes into developing the prototypes. Nevertheless, we share the speculative designers' anxieties that this way of engaging with participants is always potentially fraught. The idiocy of the probes and the prototypes might simply alienate their users, not least in those settings (offshore sites, for instance) that are material-culturally dissimilar to the home settings in which speculative design originated and developed. Here, the importance of initial ethnographic engagements with potential volunteers is even more important than usual. Having made this point, it remains the case that probes and prototypes are always chronically at risk of 'failure' – failure to engage their users' attention, interest and practical involvement.

At the risk of even greater repetition, the whole point of the collaborative process we have described is to enable inventive problem-making. On this score, let us further gloss PigeonBlog. It should be clear that it has played a part in reframing the issue of air quality measurement and control, of creatively re-inventing the 'problem of air quality'. But, further, this has been done in a way which makes the problem 'more tractable' in the sense that the problem's traction comes to be extended beyond the scientists' initial framing to address the experience and concerns of local residents. Thus, a speculative prototype ideally should generate a range of responses some of which can entail 'creative problem-making'. In the present case, we would hope to find a creative re-invention of 'the problem of HIV prevention'. Crucial to all this is the fact that this emergent 'inventive problem of HIV prevention' has emerged through participants' complex engagement with the prototype (which, it should be obvious by now, is designed to enable such complex engagement). As such, the further hope is that this emergent 'inventive problem of HIV prevention' will inform the development of policies and strategies for HIV prevention and prophylactic implementation which are more consonant with such complexity, that have greater traction in the context of such complexity.

Yet, this consonance and traction also operate in a different way. The playfulness, obliqueness, ambiguity of prototypes and probes are designed to encourage users to explore not only 'what is' but also 'what might be'. That is to say, participants' can use these devices to engage with the personal and collective virtualities that can be attached to the local eventuations of HIV prevention. This prospecting of prospects can likewise inform policy and biomedical practice – it is a resource that can alert professionals and practitioners to complex and shifting possibilities that can become manifest unexpectedly.

Of course, it would be remiss of us not apply our version of the event to the present eventuation of our interdisciplinary collaboration. Informing this is an abstraction, an attractor – at base, this presumes a sort of ease of collaboration, a happy investment in the practices of interdisciplinary work. At a more optimistic level, another attractor might frame such collaborations as an event of becoming-with: the disciplinary idiocy of speculative design thus occasions an exchange of qualities between designers, biomedical and social scientists. However, there are also likely to be lurking in the virtual a series of 'anti-attractors'. For instance, there is the well-worn potential that for all the encouragement that interdisciplinary collaboration ostensibly receives from various funding bodies, this routinely fails to translate into funding support. And of course there are the anti-attractors of the collaborators' distinct disciplines: each is likely to be drawn to addressing their home audiences.

Nevertheless, despite these potential (and other) pitfalls, there seems to be some promise in this strategy. Moreover, it does not simply apply to HIV prevention, and the 'creative re-invention' of the 'problem' of PrEP, RCTs and bioethics. It is a strategy that can apply no less to the emergence and potential use of other 'innovative health technologies' (IHTs). In dealing with the controversies that on occasion surround such emergent IHTs, one key contemporary response (especially in Western Europe and North America) is the development and application of techniques of 'public engagement with science' which generally bring laypeople and experts together in some form of dialogue (this is also allied to attempts to introduce a public voice further 'upstream' in the innovation process). There are many well-known problems with these initiatives: for instance, they presuppose a particular framing of the issues to be addressed, they ultimately serve in the muting or limiting of public voice, they are no better than public relations exercises (see Michael, 2012b). What the present advocacy for collaborations with speculative design (and, we might add, various forms of art practice) points to are ways of creatively rethinking these modes of engagement which allow for an emergent reinvention of the IHT problem at stake. The broader hope is that such a reinvention incorporates a rethinking not only of the 'nature' of the IHT in question but also what it means to be, for example, a member of the public, a user, an ethicist, a biomedical scientist, a citizen, and even a social scientist.

Notes

1 Introduction: Setting a Scene

1. The brand name for Tenofovir is Viread® (or Tenofovir Disoproxil Fumarate). The brand name for Emtricitibane is Emtriva®. Both drugs are manufactured by Gilead Sciences Inc.
2. According to a major report edited by Lagakos and Gable titled *Methodological Challenges in Biomedical HIV Prevention Trials*: 'efficacy refers to the effect of the intervention in a tightly controlled setting, wherein investigators try to minimize factors such as imperfect adherence to the product regimen, changes in risk behaviour, and changes in the risk of exposure to HIV. Effectiveness, on the other hand, refers to how well the intervention would perform in the real world, where these factors and others cannot be rigorously controlled....' (2008:75,76).
3. A guide to the principles set out in the Helsinki Declaration and the many modifications that have taken place since its first signing in 1964 (after the Nuremberg Trials in post-Nazi Germany) is available at http://www.wma.net/en/30publications/10policies/b3/ [accessed 23 November 2012].

2 A Brief and Partial History of Randomized Controlled Trials (RCTs) in the Context of HIV Prevention and Treatment

1. For full discussion on differences between Phase 1, Phase 2, Phase 2b and Phase 3 trials see chapter 2, 'Basic Design Features: Size, Duration, and Type of Trials, and Choice of Control Group' in S. W. Lagakos and A. R. Gable, (eds) (2008) *Methodological Challenges in HIV Prevention Trials* (National Academies Press) available on line: http://www.nap.edu/catalog.php?record_id=12056 (69–87).
2. An approach somewhat akin to what we are alluding to here can be found in Anita Hardon's (2006) account of how a public health strategy of population control to force women to take on long lasting contraception was challenged by a diverse but user-oriented women's health advocacy. The latter avoided direct opposition and, instead, advocated for strategies designed with user preferences as the priority. In other words, the 'script', as Hardon puts it, to capture how technologies emerge in ways that affect their users, came to involve the introduction of a range of contraceptives available for use on the basis of 'informed choice' (2006:625). Without going into the details of Hardon's work (nor how we might understand the notion of 'choice'), it is apparent that the heterogeneous elements active in the emergence of a health intervention can be affected in ways that become, in effect, what the intervention 'is' and, therefore, does.

3. For a full account see GCM (Global Campaign for Microbicides) available at: http://www.global-campaign.org/more_microbicides.htm#pregnant [accessed 30 September 2012].

4. This claim is based on one of the authors witnessing a standing ovation for the researchers at AIDS 2010 Vienna, the biannual conference for the HIV field usually attended by over 15,000 delegates.

5. According to NIAID (National Institute of Allergy and Infectious Diseases), the first HIV vaccine trial commenced in 1987 in Maryland, USA. The trial enrolled 138 uninfected research subjects. The trial tested 'gp 160 subunit vaccine'. No serious adverse effects were reported. http://www.niaid.nih. gov/topics/hivaids/research/vaccines/Pages/history.aspx [accessed 5 October 2012].

6. Researchers at the University of Washington have since found 'that antibodies specific to the V1V2 region of the HIV genome correlated with lower risk of infection'. In other words, it is suggested that the capacity of the vaccine is related to the genetic nature of the strain of virus. Thus to be effective, the vaccine had to elicit an immune response that intercepted certain genetic strains of the virus. However, the vaccine was not able to exert pressure on all the genetic variations of 'the' virus. See Nodell (2012) http://www.wash-ington.edu/news/2012/09/14/researchers-come-a-step-closer-to-finding-hiv-vaccine/ [accessed 5 October 2012].

7. The study most commonly referred to as the STEP study or Merck V520 Protocol 023/HVTN 502), randomized 3000 research subjects across two arms – a placebo and one involving the vaccine candidate.

8. Note that Zidovudine (ZDV) is also referred to as AZT. The intervention, consisting of zidovudine (ZDV) given PO [orally] to the women during the last weeks of pregnancy and IV [intraveneously] during labour and delivery, as well as to the newborns for 6 weeks, reduced the rate of infant infection from 25.5% to 8.3%. See Burr (2012).

4   The Gold Standard: The Complex Singularity of PrEP, RCT and Bioethics

1. Of course, at this stage we are simply setting out our analytic stall. However, we can mention by way of illustration that 'gold standard-ness' also concerns the nature of evidence. That is to say, the core tendency is for RCTs to enact an unqualified conception of 'evidence'. This 'evidence' (achieved through the process of singularization) serves as a measure of 'efficacy', although this is often conflated with 'effectiveness' which is intended to address 'real world' conditions. One is tempted to say that 'efficacy' and 'effectiveness' in part map respectively onto the 'quantitative' and 'qualitative' as we are using them here. However, the qualitative nature of effectiveness is still verymuch imbued with the quantitative which involves, at base, the distinction between the object (PrEP) from the user – that is, trial participant – in which these retain their separate identities rather than co-emerge or become-with in the event of the trial. The point is that while there are elements within the design of RCTs that address the qualitative,

these are routinely subverted by the recourse to the quantitative entrenched in biomedical practice.

2. Noted side-effects are nausea, diarrhoea, vomiting and intestinal gas. There is also some evidence that Tenofovir may affect the liver or kidneys in people with HIV, or result in a small decrease in bone density in some patients (see Paxton et al., 2007).

3. Assessment of post-exposure prophylaxis is difficult because in most cases it is not possible to confirm that exposure to the virus has taken place.

4. This was explained to us by one of our interviewee bench scientists. More recent evidence, however, suggests that the two drugs have different penetration capacities in relation to the walls of the vagina and the anus (see Paxton, 2012:558).

5. The likely enrolment early on in the trial of people who were not injecting drug users was suggested to us when we interviewed people associated with the trial in Bangkok in 2008.

6. The report was initiated by GCM (Global Campaign for Microbicides) and followed an earlier one on the Cameroon trial by McGrory et al. (2009). Both were prepared with the aims of providing a more informed understanding of what had brought about the opposition to PrEP trials and the lessons this might offer to the continued implementation of topical microbicide trials.

7. See for example: http://www.aidsmap.com/Trial-ethics-and-controversies /page/1746666/ [accessed 23 April 2013].

8. Up until its suspension, the Cameroon trial had ten seroconversions: six of these were in the placebo arm and four in the Tenofovir arm. The trial researchers reported that most of the women believed they had become HIV positive with their regular partners with whom they did not use a condom (McGrory et al., 2009:23). The report by McGrory et al. (2009:23) provides a comprehensive account of the negotiations that took place leading up to FHI establishing a formalized agreement for medical care with a hospital in Douala, the city where the trial was conducted.

9. Although this is a view widely accepted and for sound empirical reasons, there is evidence that the practice can be complex in ways that indicate clean needles and syringes are not all that may be required. In 2005, McCurdy reported: 'Female sex workers who inject heroin in Tanzania, have created a new needle sharing practice they call "flashblood." This entails drawing the first blood back in a syringe until the barrel is full and then passing the needle and syringe to a female companion. Women believe that about 4 cm^3 of such blood contains enough heroin to help them escape the pains of withdrawal. They developed this practice in mid-2005 in an altruistic attempt to help one another. Where water is contaminated, injectors may use blood to mix the powder of the drug as a means of producing a liquid.'

10. http://fhi.org/en/Research/Projects/FEM-PrEP.htm [accessed 6 January 2012].

11. http://fhi.org/NR/rdonlyres/erj6hevouwvddigjldvcca6tvtybfolh4nedyfe-o4yz2i7la53jknim6ex42bme2rvyq6zfzovyrkb/FEMPrEPFactSheetJune2011. pdf [accessed 6 January 2012].

12. Having ruled out what they refer to as possible cultural explanations for the doubling of HIV incidence in pregnant women, Gray et al. (2005) suggest that the cause may lie with hormonal factors affecting changes at a cellular

level where the virus gains entry or exploits changes to the immune system induced by the presence of a foetus.

5 PrEPs, Multiplicity and the Qualification of Knowledge and Ethics

1. The inverted commas connote the fact that these are terms typical of the standard accounts of RCTs, but which we are, it should be obvious, intent on troubling: at the very least, each is implicated in the others.
2. According to Padian et al. (2010:631), unexpectedly low rates of HIV incidence occurred in 14 (64 per cent) of 22 prevention RCTs, hence no significant differences between the randomized trial arms could be claimed; this was similarly the case in one PrEP study in Botswana (cited in Chapter 2) and consequently it became impracticable to evaluate efficacy.
3. GCM (The Global Campaign for Microbicides) offers the following explanation for why topical vaginal microbicides are needed for women: 'Today's prevention options – condoms, mutual monogamy, and STI treatment – are not feasible for millions of people around the world, especially women. Many women do not have the social or economic power necessary to insist on condom use and fidelity or to abandon partnerships that put them at risk. Because microbicides would not require a partner's cooperation, they would put the power to protect into women's hands'. http://www.global-campaign. org/about_microbicides.htm [accessed 23 November 2012].
4. CDC 'Pre-Exposure Prophylaxis (PrEP)' http://www.cdc.gov/hiv/prep/ [accessed 7 January 2012].
5. FHI (Family Health International) FEM-PrEP fact sheet June 2011 update http://fhi.org/NR/rdonlyres/erj6hevouwvddigjldvcca6tvtybfolh4nedyfe-o4yz2i7la53jknim6ex42bme2rvyq6zfzovyrkb/FEMPrEPFactSheetJune2011. pdf [accessed 6 January 2012].
6. The WNU (Women's Network for Unity) is a non-government organization run by a union of Cambodian sex workers. According to the Global Campaign for Microbicides (2009:8) 'The organising efforts that led to its creation began in 1997'. They go on to quote material produced by the WNU to explain its purpose as follows: 'It provides a foundation for support and builds solidarity and self empowerment among sex workers. Our network provides a space for women to come together, share ideas and discuss the collective challenges we face.'

6 On Some Topologies of PrEP

1. URL (Consulted last accessed 12 May 2011) http://mathworld.wolfram.com/ Topology.html.
2. http://www.unaids.org/en/aboutunaids/ [accessed 8 September 2012].
3. Not surprising but indicative of the complex network of relations that exist within the HIV assemblage, it is apparent that UNAIDS and WHO reports most usually involve a list of participants that may include large non-government organizations such as AVAC (Aids Advocacy Coalition)

which receives a substantial amount of funding for its work from the Bill and Melinda Gates Foundation which is also the main philanthropic funder of HIV biomedical prevention RCTs, including those for PrEP. Consultations may include representatives of government health ministries in countries with high HIV prevalence such as Uganda and South Africa. They may also include well-known epidemiologists from low income countries such Peru who may, in turn, also be members of the governing council of the International AIDS Society.

4. Although we also note that the trial referred to continues to be regarded as highly contentious by some (see, for example, Craddock, 2004)
5. URL (accessed 9 April 2010) http://www.opendoorcli nic.org/.
6. See United States Leadership Against HIV/AIDS, Tuberculosis, and Malaria Act of 2003. http://www.avert.org/pepfar.htm#contentTable3 [accessed 2 April 2012].
7. It is worth noting that the moralism evident in PEPFAR funding policies reflects the longstanding postures toward HIV within the United States. See Global Campaign for Microbicides, 2009:10.
8. Here we would like to thank Kane Race for drawing our attention to the work of Neville Hoad.

7   Conclusion: Eventuating the Methodology of Trials

1. http://www.fda.gov/NewsEvents/Newsroom/PressAnnouncements /ucm312210.htm [accessed 5 November 2012].
2. The same claim was made in a report issued by UNAIDS (2012) titled 'Together we will end AIDS' published by the Joint United Nations Programme on HIV /AIDS (UNAIDS)
3. The CDC trial conducted in Botswana called TDF2 was initially part of a multi-site trial including Nigeria and Malawi. However only Botswana went ahead, due to what were reported as logistical difficulties in Nigeria and Malawi (there was no reporting of any controversy about the ethics of these). The Botswana trial (on young adult heterosexual men and women between the ages of 18 and 39 who were recruited in Gaborone and Francistown initially to test oral Tenofovir though this was changed to the anticipated more efficacious Truvada) was initially regarded as too small to provide efficacy data and thus it was continued as a safety trial. However, although it was not mentioned as a contributor to impending efficacy results in publications up to 2011, in light of the release of findings on the use of Truvada in the Partners PrEP study (in which CDC was also involved), CDC released their Botswana findings earlier than planned. It presented the Botswana study as further evidence of PrEP having a protective effect in heterosexual sex (CDC, 2011) and, of special note, that PrEP offered a protective effect in women. The evidence of PrEP's efficacy in women was particularly important and enabling of FDA approval given the failure of the Fem-PrEP RCT to demonstrate PrEP efficacy in women (see Chapter 4).
4. The term 'demonstration study' is now used widely but without specification so it is difficult to offer a more precise account of what such a study could

involve (see, for example, WHO, 2012b). What is evident is that these studies are intended to shed light on the effects of taking PrEP outside an efficacy study.

5. An outline of the design research ethos behind the Interaction Research Studio and examples of various prototypes and techniques can be found at; http://www.gold.ac.uk/interaction/public/ [accessed 7 November 2012].

Glossary

ACT UP The AIDS Coalition to Unleash Power mostly active in the period prior to the introduction of antiretroviral therapy.

ACTG 076 RCT randomized, double-blind, controlled clinical trial of zidovudine (AZT) for reducing the rate of transmission from mother to infant implemented in United States.

AIDS Acquired Immunodeficiency Syndrome.

ALVAC-AIDSVAX (RV 144) vaccine RCT conducted in Thailand.

ARV antiretroviral drugs for suppressing the replication of HIV in vivo.

AVAC AIDS Vaccine Advocacy Coalition.

AZT zidovudine (formerly azidothymidine) also termed ACTG 076.

BMGF Bill and Melinda Gates Foundation.

CAPRISA or CAPRISA 004 double-blind, randomized, controlled microbicide trial of a 1% tenofovir gel in women implemented in Durban and Vulindlela in KwaZulu-Natal, South Africa.

CDC US Centers for Disease Control and Prevention.

CDC 4370 double-blind, randomized, controlled PrEP trial of daily Tenofovir-Disoproxil Fumarate (TDF) in Injection Drug Users in Bangkok, Thailand.

CHAMP The Community HIV/AIDS Mobilisation Project.

COL-1492 nonoxynol-9 RCT.

Emtricitabine also called FTC, an antiretroviral drug in the class of nucleotide analogue reverse transcriptase inhibitors (NRTIs).

FDA United States of America Food and Drug Administration.

FEM-PrEP randomized, double-blinded, placebo-controlled trial of once-daily oral co-formulated emtricitabine/tenofovir disoproxil fumarate (FTC/TDF) implemented in South Africa, Kenya and Tanzania.

FHI Family Health International.

FTC emtricitabine, an antiretroviral drug in the class of nucleotide analogue reverse transcriptase (NRTIs).

GCM Global Campaign for Microbicides.

GRID gay-related immune deficiency which was the initial biomedical name given to HIV.

HIV human immunodeficiency virus.

HVTN HIV Vaccines Trials Network.

IAS International AIDS Society.

IAVI International AIDS Vaccine Initiative.

IDUs Injecting Drug Users.

iPrEX double-blinded, placebo-controlled trial of once-daily oral co-formulated emtricitabine/tenofovir disoproxil fumarate (FTC/TDF) implemented in men who have sex with men (MSM) and transgender women in Peru, Ecuador, South Africa, Brazil, Thailand, and the United States.

MIRA RCT Methods for Improving Reproductive Health in Africa assessed whether a package including the diaphragm and condom was more efficacious against HIV than condoms.

MSM men who have sex with men.

MTN Microbicides Trials Network.

NGO nongovernmental organization.

Nonoxynol-9 vaginal spermicide.

NIH US National Institutes of Health.

Partners PrEP randomized, double-blinded, placebo-controlled trial of once-daily oral tenofovir arm and a once-daily oral co-formulated emtricitabine/tenofovir disoproxil fumarate (FTC/TDF) arm implemented in females and males in sero-discordant regular relationships in Kenya and Uganda.

PrEP pre-exposure prophylaxis.

PEPFAR President's Emergency Plan for AIDS.

REDS Réseau Ethique Droit et Santé (Network for Ethics, Laws, and Health)

Sero-discordant where one partner has HIV and the other does not have HIV.

TDF tenofovir disoproxil fumarate or Viread, an antiretroviral drug in the class of nucleotide analogue reverse transcriptase (NRTIs).

TDF2 PrEP RCT randomized, double-blinded, placebo-controlled trial of once daily oral TDF/FTC (Truvada) to reduce HIV infection in both men and women implanted in Botswana.

Tenofovir disoproxil fumarate also referred to as TDF or Viread, an antiretroviral drug in the class of nucleotide analogue reverse transcriptase inhibitors (NRTIs).

Topical microbicide a gel, suppository or cream inserted into the vagina or rectum to prevent HIV can be contrasted with a systemic oral preparation such as Truvada which is ingested.

Truvada TDF and FTC both antiretroviral drugs in the class of nucleotide analogue reverse transcriptase inhibitors (NRTIs) combined in one pill.

UNAIDS Joint United Nations Programme on HIV/AIDS.

UNFPA United Nations Population Fund.

USAID United States of America Aid.

VOICE Vaginal and Oral Interventions to Control the Epidemic randomized, double-blinded, placebo-controlled trial of once-daily tenofovir arm and a once-daily oral co-formulated emtricitabine/tenofovir disoproxil fumarate (FTC/TDF) arm plus an arm with Tenofovir vaginal topical microbicide implemented in women in South Africa, Uganda and Zimbabwe.

WHO World Health Organization.

Zidovudine (ZDV) also referred to as AZT.

Bibliography

U.L. Abbas, R.M. Anderson and J. W. Mellors (2007) 'Potential Impact of Antiretroviral Chemoprophylaxis on HIV-1 Transmission in Resource-Limited Settings', *PLos One* 9:e875: 1–11, available at www.plosone.org [accessed 16 November 2012].

Q. Abdool Karim et al. (2010) 'Effectiveness and Safety of Tenofovir Gel, an Antiretroviral Microbicide, for the Prevention of HIV Infection in Women' *Science* 329:1168–74.

B. Adam (2011) 'Epistemic Fault Lines in Biomedical and Social Approaches to HIV Prevention', *Journal of the International AIDS Society* 14(Suppl 2):S2.

AIDSMAP (2012) http://www.aidsmap.com/en/Email-a friend/tpl/1412195 /page/2278778/ [accessed 20 March 2012].

M. Akrich (1992) 'The De-scription of Technical Objects' in W.E. Bijker and J. Law (eds) *Shaping Technology/Building Society* (Cambridge, MA: MIT Press).

M. Angell (2000) 'Investigators' Responsibilities for Human Subjects in Developing Countries', *New England Journal Of Medicine* 342,13:967–9.

K. Ansell Pearson (1999) *Germinal Life* (London: Routledge).

H. Arksey (1998) *RSI and the Experts: The Construction of Medical Knowledge* (London: UCL Press).

J. D. Auerbach and T.J. Coates (2000) 'HIV Prevention Research: Accomplishments and Challenges for the Third Decade of AIDS', *American Journal of Public Health* 90:1029–32.

J.D. Auerbach et al. (2011) 'Addressing Social Drivers of HIV/AIDS for the Long-term Response: Conceptual and Methodological Considerations', *Global Public Health* 6 Suppl 3:S293–309.

AVAC (AIDS Vaccine Advocacy Coalition) (2005) *Will a Pill a Day Prevent HIV? Anticipating the Results of 'PREP' Trials* (New York: AVAC).

AVAC (2008) *Anticipating the Results of PrEP Trials: A Powerful New HIV Prevention Tool May Be on the Horizon.* A publication from AVAC's *Anticipating and Understanding Results* series August 2008.

AVAC (2011) http://www.avac.org/ht/display/ReleaseDetails/i/33409/pid/212%20 cited%204%20August%202011 [accessed 19 February 2013].

AVAC (2013) http://data.avac.org/OngoingPrepTrials.aspx [accessed 19 February 2013].

J.M. Baeten et al. (2012) 'Antiretroviral Prophylaxis for HIV Prevention in Heterosexual Men and Women', *New England Journal of Medicine* 367:399–410.

K. Barad (1998) 'Getting Real: Technoscientific Practices and the Materialization of Reality', *Differences: A Journal of Feminist Cultural Studies* 10, 2:87–128.

K. Barad (2007) *Meeting the Universe Halfway* (Durham, NC: Duke University Press).

B. Barnes (1977) *Interests and the Growth of Knowledge* (London: RKP).

T. Barnighausen, J.A. Salomon and N. Sangrujee (2012) 'HIV Treatment as Prevention: Issues in Economic Evaluation', *PLoS Medicine* 1 July 2012 9, 7: e1001263, available at www.plosmedicine.org [accessed 6 August 2012].

A. Barry (2001) *Political Machines* (London: Athlone).

A. Barry (2005) 'Pharmaceutical Matters: The Invention of Informed Materials', *Theory, Culture and Society* 22(1):51–69.

A. Barry, G. Born and G. Weszkalnys (2008) 'Logics of Interdisciplinarity', *Economy and Society* 37:20–49.

E. Bass and P. Kahn (2005) 'Testing AIDS Vaccines in People' in P. Kahn (ed.) *AIDS Vaccine Handbook: Global Perspectives*, 2nd edn (New York: AVAC).

F. Beckman (2009) 'The Idiocy of the Event: Between Antonin Artaud, Kathy Acker and Gilles Deleuze', *Deleuze Studies* 3(1):54–72.

S. Beder (1999) 'Public Participation or Public Relations' in B. Martin (ed.) *Technology and Public Participation* (pp. 169–292) (Wollongong, Australia: Science and Technology Studies, University of Wollongong).

J. Bennett (2010) *Vibrant Matter* (Durham, NC: Duke University Press).

W.E. Bijker (1995) *Of Bicycles, Bakelite and Bulbs: Toward a Theory of Sociotechnical Change* (Cambridge, MA: The MIT Press).

D. Bloor (1976) *Knowledge and Social Imagery* (London: RKP).

K. Boehner, W. Gaver and A. Boucher (2012) 'Probes' in C. Lury and N. Wakeford (eds) *Inventive Methods: The Happening of the Social* (London: Routledge).

G. Born and A. Barry (2010) '"ART-SCIENCE": From Public Understanding to Public Experiment', *Journal of Cultural Economy* 3:103–19.

M. Borup et al. (2006) 'The Sociology of Expectations in Science and Technology', *Technology Analysis & Strategic Management*, 18:285–98.

K. Braun and S. Schultz (2010) '"...a certain amount of engineering involved": Constructing the Public in Participatory Governance Arrangements', *Public Understanding of Science* 19:403–19.

N. Brown (2003) 'Hope Against Hype – Accountability in Biopasts, Presents and Futures', *Science Studies* 16:3–21.

N. Brown and M. Michael (2003) 'A Sociology of Expectations: Retrospecting Prospects and Prospecting Retrospects', *Technology Analysis and Strategic Management* 15:3–18.

N. Brown and A. Webster (2004) *New Medical Technologies and Society: Reordering Life* (Cambridge: Polity).

N. Brown, B. Rappert and A. Webster (eds) (2000) *Contested Futures* (Aldershot: Ashgate).

C.K. Burr (2012) 'Reducing Perinatal HIV Transmission: Guide for HIV/AIDS Clinical Care' HRSA HIV/AIDS Bureau, available at: http://www.aidsetc.org/aidsetc?page=cg-402_pmtct [accessed 9 November 2012).

D.P. Byar et al. (1990) 'Design Considerations for AIDS Trials', *New England Journal of Medicine* 323:1343–8.

D. Callahan (1999) 'The Social Sciences and the Task of Bioethics', *Daedalus* 128:275–94.

M. Callon and B. Latour (1981) 'Unscrewing the Big Leviathan' in K.D. Knorr-Cetina and M. Mulkay (eds) *Advances in Social Theory and Methodology* (London: Routledge and Kegan Paul).

M. Callon and J. Law (1982) 'On Interests and Their Transformation: Enrolment and Counter-Enrolment', *Social Studies of Science* 12:615–25.

M. Callon (1986a) 'The Sociology of an Actor-Network: The Case of the Electric Vehicle' in M. Callon, J. Law and A. Rip (eds) *Mapping the Dynamics of Science and Technology* (London: Macmillan).

M. Callon (1986b) 'Some Elements in a Sociology of Translation: Domestication of the Scallops and Fishermen of St Brieuc Bay' in J. Law (ed.) *Action and Belief* (London: Routledge and Kegan Paul).

M. Callon, P. Lascoumbes and Y. Barthe (2001) *Acting in an Uncertain World: An Essay on Technical Democracy* (Cambridge, MA: The MIT Press).

M. Callon and V. Rabeharisoa (2008) 'The Growing Engagement of Emergent Concerned Groups in Political and Economic Life: Lessons from the French Association of Neuromuscular Disease Patients', *Science, Technology, and Human Values* 33:230–61.

M.M. Cassell et al. (2006) 'Risk Compensation: the Achilles' Heel of Innovations in HIV Prevention?', *British Medical Journal* 332:605–7.

CDC (2011) http://www.cdc.gov/nchhstp/newsroom/PrEPHeterosexuals.html [accessed 10 November 2012].

CDC (2012) 'Pre-Exposure Prophylaxis (PrEP)' http://www.cdc.gov/hiv/prep/ [accessed 7 January 2012].

M.S. Cohen et al. (2011) 'Prevention of HIV-1 Infection with Early Antiretroviral Therapy', *New England Journal of Medicine* 365:493–505.

M.S. Cohen and L.R. Baden (2012) 'Preexposure Prophylaxis for HIV — Where Do We Go from Here?', *New England Medical Journal* 367 (5):459,460.

H.M. Collins (1985) *Changing Order* (London: Sage).

M. Cooper (2011) 'Trial by Accident: Tort Law, Industrial Risks and the History of Medical Experiment', *Journal of Cultural Economy* 4(1):81–96.

R.S. Cowan (1987) 'The Consumption Junction: A Proposal for Research Strategies in the Sociology of Technology' in W.E. Bijker, T.P. Hughes and T. Pinch (eds) *Social Construction of Technological Systems* (Cambridge, MA: MIT Press).

S. Craddock (2004) 'AIDS and Ethics: Clinical Trials, Pharmaceuticals, and Global Scientific Practice' in E. Kalipeni, S. Craddock, J.R. Oppong and J. Ghosh (eds) *HIV & AIDS in Africa: Beyond Epidemiology* (Maldon, USA, Oxford UK, Victoria, Australia: Blackwell Publishing).

G. Davies (2006) 'Mapping Deliberation: Calculation, Articulation and Intervention in the Politics of Organ Transplantation', *Economy and Society* 35:232–58.

M. DeLanda (2002) *Intensive Science and Virtual Philosophy* (London: Continuum).

G. Deleuze (2004) *Difference and Repetition* (London: Continuum).

G. Deleuze and F. Guattari (1988) *A Thousand Plateaus: Capitalism and Schizophrenia* (London: Athlone Press).

G. Deleuze and F.Guattari (1994) *What is Philosophy?* (London: Verso).

I. Derdelinckx et al. (2006) 'Criteria for Drugs Used in Pre-Exposure Prophylaxis Trials against HIV Infection', *PloS Medicine* 11, e454 0001–6.

P. de Zulueta (2001) 'Randomised Placebo-Controlled Trials and HIV-Infected Pregnant Women in Developing Countries. Ethical Imperialism or Unethical Exploitation?', *Bioethics* 15(4):291–311.

G.W. Dowsett and M. Couch (2007) 'Male Circumcision and HIV Prevention: Is There Really Enough of the Right Kind of Evidence?', *Reproductive Health Matters*, 15(29):33–44.

J.B. Dumond et al. (2007) 'Antiretroviral Drug Exposure in the Female Genital Tract: Implications for Oral Pre- and Post-exposure Prophylaxis', *AIDS* 21:1899–907.

J.W. Eaten et al. (2012) 'HIV Treatment as Prevention: Systematic Comparison of Mathematical Models of the Potential Impact of Antiretroviral Therapy on HIV

Incidence in South Africa', *PLOS Medicine* July. Online publication, available at: http://www.plosmedicine.org/article/info%3Adoi%2F10.1371%2Fjournal.pmed.1001245 [accessed 6 October 2012].

M. Elam and M. Bertilsson (2003) 'Consuming, Engaging and Confronting Science: The Emerging Dimensions of Scientific Citizenship', *European Journal of Social Theory* 6:233–51.

D. Elliot (2011) 'Imagining "Atlanta": Spatiality and the cultural politics of experimental medicine in East Africa,' paper given at *Locating the Social: 1st International Humanities and Social Science Conference*, 11–13 June 2011 in Durban, South Africa.

N. Emmerich (2011) 'Literature, History and the Humanization of Bioethics', *Bioethics* 25:112–18.

S. Epstein (1996) *Impure Science: AIDS Activism and the Politics of Science* (Berkeley, CA: University of California Press).

S. Epstein (2004) 'Bodily Differences and Collective Identities: The Politics of Gender and Race in Biomedical Research in the United States', *Body and Society* 10 (2–3):183–203.

J.H. Evans (2006) 'Between Technocracy and Democratic Legitimation: A Proposed Compromise Position for Common Morality Public Bioethics', *Journal of Medicine and Philosophy* 31:213–34.

U. Felt et al. (2009) 'Unruly Ethics: On the Difficulties of a Bottom-up Approach to Ethics in the Field of Genomics', *Public Understanding of Science* 18:354–71.

P. Flowers (2001) 'Gay Men and HIV/AIDS Risk Management', *Health* 5:50–75.

M. Fraser (2009) 'Standards, Populations, and Difference', *Cultural Critique* 71, Winter:47–80.

M. Fraser (2010) 'Facts, Ethics and Event' in C. Bruun Jensen and K. Rødje (eds) *Deleuzian Intersections in Science, Technology and Anthropology* (pp. 57–82) (New York, NY: Berghahn Press).

B. Freedman (1987) 'Equipoise and the Ethics of Clinical Research', *The New England Journal of Medicine* 317:141–5.

S. Fuller (2005) 'Is STS Revolutionary or Merely Revolting?', *Science Studies* 18:75–83.

S.O. Funtowitz and J. Ravetz (1993) 'Science for the Post-normal Age', *Futures* 25:739–55.

F.W. Geels (2004) 'From Sectoral Systems of Innovation to Socio-technical Systems: Insights about Dynamics and Change from Sociology and Institutional Theory', *Research Policy* 33:897–920.

GCM (Global Campaign for Microbicides) (2009) *Preventing Prevention Trial Failures: A Case Study and Lessons for Future Trials from the 2004 Tenofovir Trial in Cambodia*. Washington DC: Global Campaign for Microbicides at PATH, Program for Appropriate Technology in Health (PATH).

GCM (Global Campaign for Microbicides) available at: http://www.global-campaign.org/more_microbicides.htm#pregnant [accessed 30 September 2012].

B. Godin (2006) 'The Linear Model of Innovation: The Historical Construction of an Analytical Framework', *Science, Technology and Human Values* 31:639–67.

H. Gottweis, B. Salter and C. Waldby (2009) *The Global Politics of Human Embryonic Stem Cell Science: Regenerative Medicine in Transition* (Basingstoke: Palgrave Macmillan).

D. Grant and E. Bass (2010) 'Understanding the results of RV144, the Thai prime-boost AIDS vaccine trial', available at: http://www.avac.org/ht/d/sp/a/ GetDocumentAction/i/6328 [accessed 4 August 2011].

R.M. Grant et al. (2010) 'Preexposure Chemoprophylaxis for HIV Prevention in Men Who Have Sex with Men', *The New England Journal of Medicine* 363 (27):2587–99.

R. Gray et al. (2005) 'Increased Risk of Incident HIV during Pregnancy in Rakai, Uganda: A Prospective Study', *The Lancet* 366 (9492):1182–8.

R.M. Green, A. Donovan and S.A. Jeuss (eds) (2008) *Global Bioethics* (Oxford: Oxford University Press).

B.G. Haire (2011) 'Because We Can: Clashes of Perspective over Researcher Obligation in the Failed Prep Trials', *Developing World Bioethics* 11 (2):63–74.

M. Halewood (2011) *A Culture of Thought. A.N. Whitehead and Social Theory* (London: Anthem Press).

M. Halewood and M. Michael (2008) 'Being a Sociologist and Becoming a Whiteheadian: Concrescing Methodological Tactics', *Theory, Culture and Society* 25, 4:31–56.

D. Haraway (1997) *Modest_Witness@Second_Millenium.FemaleMan. Meets_ OncoMouse: Feminism and Technoscience* (London: Routledge).

A. Hardon (2006) 'Contesting Contraceptive Innovation – Reinventing the Script', *Social Science & Medicine* 62:614–27.

R. Harré (ed.) (1986) *The Social Construction of Emotions* (Oxford: Blackwell).

A. Hedgecoe (2010) 'Bioethics and the Reinforcement of Socio-technical Expectations', *Social Studies of Science* 40:163–86.

R. Heffron et al. (2012) 'Use of Hormonal Contraceptives and Risk of HIV-1 Transmission: A Prospective Cohort Study', *The Lancet Infectious Diseases* 12 (1):19–26.

L. Heise et al. (2011) 'Apples and Oranges? Interpreting Success in HIV Prevention Trials', *Contraception* 83:10–15.

B. Highmore (2011) *Ordinary Lives* (London: Routledge).

N. Hoad (2010) 'Three Poems and a Pandemic' in J. Staiger, A. Cvetkovich and A. Reynolds (eds) *Political Emotions: New Agendas in Communication* (pp. 134–50) (New York and London: Routledge).

D.R. Holtgrave et al. (2012) 'Behavioral Factors in Assessing Impact of HIV Treatment as Prevention', *AIDS and Behavior* 16(5):1085–91.

House of Lords Select Committee on Science and Technology (February 2000) *3rd Report: Science and Society. HL Paper 38* (London: The Stationery Office).

Human Rights Watch Thailand (2004) 'Not Enough Graves: The War on Drugs, HIV/AIDS, and Violations of Human Rights' June 2004, Vol. 16, No. 8 (C).

C.B. Hurt, J.J. Jr. Eron and M.S. Cohen (2011) 'Pre-Exposure Prophylaxis an Antiretroviral Resistance: HIV Prevention at a Cost?', *Clinical Infectious Diseases* 53:1265–70.

IAS (International AIDS Society) (2005) *Building Collaboration to Advance HIV Prevention. Global Consultation on Tenofovir Pre-Exposure Prophylaxis Research.* Report of a Consultation Convened by the International Aids Society on Behalf of the Bill and Melinda Gates Foundation US National Institutes of Health and US Centers for Disease Control and Prevention, September.

IAVI (International AIDS Vaccine Initiative) (2012) http://www.iavi.org/Who-We-Are/ Experts/Studies/Clinical-Trials/Pages/default.aspx [accessed 5 October 2012].

A. Irwin (1995) *Citizen Science: A Study of People, Expertise and Sustainable Development* (London: Routledge).

A. Irwin (2001) 'Constructing the Scientific Citizen: Science and Democracy in the Biosciences', *Public Understanding of Science* 10(1):1–18.

A. Irwin and M. Michael (2003) *Science, Social Theory and Public Knowledge* (Maidenhead, Berks: Open University Press/McGraw-Hill).

A. Irwin and B. Wynne (eds) (1996) *Misunderstanding Science? The Public Reconstruction of Science and Technology* (Cambridge: Cambridge University Press).

S. Jintarkanon et al. (2005) 'Unethical Clinical Trials in Thailand: A Community Response', *Lancet* 365:1617–18.

P-B. Joly, A. Rip and M. Callon (2010) 'Reinventing Innovation' in M. Arentsen, W. van Rossum and B. Steenge (eds) *Governance of Innovation* (pp. 19–32) (Cheltenham: Edward Elgar).

P. Kahn (ed.) (2005) *AIDS Vaccine Handbook: Global Perspectives*, 2nd edn. (New York: AVAC).

T.J. Kaptchuk (2001) 'The Double-blind, Randomized, Placebo-controlled Trial: Gold Standard or Golden Calf?', *Journal of Clinical Epidemiology* 54(6):541–9.

P. Keating and A. Cambrosio (2003) *Biomedical Platforms. Realigning the Normal and the Pathological in Late-Twentieth-Century Medicine* (Cambridge, MA: MIT Press).

S. Kippax (2003) 'Sexual Health Interventions Are Unsuitable for Experimental Evaluation' in J.M. Stephenson, J. Imrie and C. Bonell (eds) *Effective Sexual Health Interventions: Issues in Experimental Evaluation* (pp. 17–34) (Oxford: Oxford University Press).

S. Kippax (2010) 'HIV-treatment as prevention: the exclusion of the social', invited paper at the HIV and Social Exclusion seminar at the Institute for Medical Anthropology and Medical History, University of Oslo in collaboration with the Norwegian Directorate of Health, Oslo: 18th June.

S. Kippax (2011) 'The social barriers to effective HIV prevention', paper given at *6th International AIDS Society Conference on HIV Pathogenesis* 17–20 July, Rome, Italy.

S. Kippax and K. Race (2003) 'Sustaining Safe Practice: Twenty Years On', *Social Science & Medicine* 57:1–12.

S. Kippax and M. Holt (2009) *The State of Social and Political Science Research Related to HIV: A Report for the International AIDS Society* (Geneva: International AIDS Society).

S. Kippax, M. Holt and S. R. Friedman (2011) 'Bridging the Social and the Biomedical: Engaging the Social and Political Sciences in HIV Research', *Journal of the International AIDS Society* 14(Suppl 2):S1

S. Kippax and N. Stephenson (2012) *American Journal of Public Health* 102, 5:789–99.

S.W. Lagakos and A.R. Gable (eds) (2008) *Methodological Challenges in HIV Prevention Trials* (National Academies Press), available online at: http://www.nap.edu/catalog.php?record_id=12056 [accessed 5 January 2013].

S. Lash and C. Lury (2007) *Global Culture Industry: The Mediation of Things* (Cambridge: Polity).

B. Latour (1987) *Science in Action: How to Follow Engineers in Society* (Milton Keynes: Open University Press).

B. Latour (2005) *Reassembling the Social: An Introduction to Actor-Network-Theory* (Oxford: Oxford University Press).

J. Law (2004) *After Method: Mess in Social Science Research* (London: Routledge).

J. Law and J. Hassard (eds) (1999) *Actor Network and After* (Oxford and Keele: Blackwell and the Sociological Review).

J. Law and V. Singleton (in press) 'ANT and Politics: Working in and on the World', *Qualitative Sociology*.

N. Lee and S. Brown (1994) 'Otherness and Actor Network: The Undiscovered Continent', *American Behavioral Scientist* 37:772–90.

A.J. London (2007) 'Clinical Equipoise: Foundational Requirement or Fundamental Error?' in B. Steinbock (ed.) *The Oxford Handbook of Bioethics* (pp. 571–96) (New York: Oxford University Press).

P. Lurie and S. Wolfe (1997) 'Unethical Trials of Interventions to Reduce Perinatal Transmission of the Human Immunodeficiency Virus in Developing Countries', *The New England Journal of Medicine* 337 (12):853–6.

C. Lury, L. Parisi and T. Terranova (eds) (2012) 'Introduction: The Becoming Topological of Culture', *Theory Culture and Society* 29:3–35.

M. Lynch (1985) *Art and Artifact in Laboratory Science* (London: Routledge and Kegan Paul).

S.A McCurdy et al. (2005) 'New Injecting Practice Increases HIV Risk among Drug Users in Tanzania', available online at: *British Medical Journal* 331 doi: http://dx.doi.org/10.1136/bmj.331.7519.778-a (published 29 September 2005).

E. McGrory, A. Irvin and L. Heise (2009) *Research Rashomon: Lessons from the Cameroon Pre-exposure Prophylaxis Trial Site* (Washington DC: Global Campaign for Microbicides at PATH).

K.M. MacQueen (2011) 'Framing the Social in Biomedical HIV Prevention Trials: A 20-year Retrospective', *Journal International AIDS Society* 14(Suppl 2):S3.

K.M. MacQueen et al. HPTN 035 Standard Of Care Assessment Team (2007) 'Community Perspectives on Care Options for HIV Prevention Trial Participants', *AIDS Care* 19 (4):554–60.

N. Marres and L. McGoey (2012) 'Experimental failure: Notes on the limits of the performativity of markets', available online at http://www.academia.edu/2069737/Experimental_failure_Notes_on_the_limits_of_the_performativity_of_markets_with_L_McGoey_[accessed 19 February 2013].

E. Martin (1998) 'Anthropology and Cultural Study of Science', *Science Technology and Human Values* 23: 24–44.

B. Massumi (2002) *Parables of the Virtual* (Durham, NC: Duke University Press).

S.N. Mavedzenge et al. (2011) 'Determinants of Differential HIV Incidence among Women in Three Southern African Locations', *Journal of Acquired Immune Deficiency Syndrome* 58(1):89–99.

S. Rozario et al. (2012) 'Exploring research participants' perceptions and comprehension of the informed consent process in a pre-exposure HIV prevention study: a case study' Poster Presentation AIDS Vaccine 2012, 9–12 September. http://www.retrovirology.com/content/pdf/1742–4690-9-S2-P238.pdf [accessed 23 November 2012].

M. Michael (1992) 'Lay Discourses of Science: Science-in-General, Science-in-Particular and Self' Science', *Technology and Human Values* 17:313–33.

M. Michael (2000) *Reconnecting Culture, Technology and Nature: From Society to Heterogeneity* (London: Routledge).

M. Michael (2006) *Technoscience and Everyday Life* (Maidenhead, Berks: Open University Press/McGraw-Hill).

M. Michael (2011) 'Affecting the Technoscientific Body: Stem Cells, Wheeled-Luggage and Emotion', *Tecnoscienza: Italian Journal of Science and Technology Studies* 2(1):53–63.

M. Michael (2012a). '"What are we busy doing?" Engaging the Idiot', *Science, Technology and Human Values* 37 (5):528–54.

M. Michael (2012b) 'Toward an Idiotic Methodology: De-signing the Object of Sociology', *The Sociological Review* 60 issue Supplement S1:166–83.

M. Michael and L. Birke (1994) 'Animal Experimentation: Enrolling the Core Set', *Social Studies of Science* 24(1):81–95.

M. Michael and N. Brown (2005) 'Scientific Citizenships: Self-Representations of Xenotransplantation's Publics', *Science as Culture* 14:38–57.

M. Michael and W. Gaver (2009) 'Home beyond Home: Dwelling with Threshold Devices', *Space and Culture* 12:359–70.

M. Michael and M. Rosengarten (2012a) 'HIV, Globalization and Topology: Of Prepositions and Propositions', *Theory, Culture & Society* 29:1–24.

M. Michael and M. Rosengarten (2012b) 'Medicine: Experimentation, Politics, Emergent Bodies', *Body and Society* 18 (3–4):1–17.

M. Michael and M. Rosengarten (in press) 'Quantitative Objects and Qualitative Things: Ethics and HIV Biomedical Prevention' in E. Casella et al. (eds) *Objects and Materials: A Routledge Companion* (London: Routledge).

M. Michael et al. (2007) 'From Core Set to Assemblage: On the Dynamics of Exclusion and Inclusion in the Failure to Derive Beta Cells from Embryonic Stem Cells', *Science Studies* 20(1):5–25.

MTN (Microbicide Trials Network) (2012) Statement on decision to discontinue use of Tenofovir Gel in VOICE, a major HIV prevention study in women, available online at: http://www.mtnstopshiv.org/node/3909 [accessed 17 November 2012].

E. Mills et al (2005a) 'Designing Research in Vulnerable Populations: Lessons from HIV Prevention Trials That Stopped Early', *British Medical Journal* 331:1403–6.

E. Mills et al. (2005b) 'Media Reporting of Tenofovir Trials in Cambodia and Cameroon', *BMC International Health and Human Rights* 5(6):2–7.

A. Mol (2002) *The Body Multiple. Ontology in Medical Practice* (Durham, NC: Duke University Press).

A. Mol and J. Law (1994) 'Regions, Networks and Fluids: Anaemia and Social Topology', *Social Studies of Science* 24:641–71.

J.S.G. Montaner et al. (2006) 'The Case for Expanding Access to Highly Active Antiretroviral Therapy to Curb the Growth of the HIV Epidemic', *Lancet* 368:531–6.

E. Mykhalovskiy and M. Rosengarten (2009) 'Introduction' in Special Issue on HIV/AIDS in its third decade: renewed critique in social and cultural analysis, *Social Theory & Health* 7(3):187–95.

E. Mykhalovskiy and L.Weir (2004) 'The Problem of Evidence-based Medicine: Directions for Social Science', *Social Science and Medicine* 59:1059–69.

Network of Sex Work Projects (2006) © 2006 Niesha Studio http://blip.tv/sexworkerspresent/taking-the-pledge-185356 [accessed 7 July 2012].

V. Nguyen et al. (2011) 'Remedicalizing an Epidemic: From HIV Treatment as Prevention to HIV Treatment Is Prevention', *AIDS* 25:291–3.

NIAID (National Institute of Allergy and Infectious Diseases) Available online at: http://www.niaid.nih.gov/topics/hivaids/research/vaccines/Pages/history.aspx [accessed 5 October 2012].

B. Nodell (2012) 'Researchers come a step closer to finding HIV vaccine', available online at: http://www.washington.edu/news/2012/09/14/researchers-come-a-step-closer-to-finding-hiv-vaccine/ [accessed 5 October 2012].

H. Nowotny, P. Scott and M. Gibbons (2001) *Re-Thinking Science: Knowledge and the Public in an Age of Uncertainty* (Cambridge: Polity).

J.J. O'Hagan et al. (2012) 'Apparent Declining Efficacy in Randomized Trials: Examples of the Thai RV144 HIV Vaccine and South African CAPRISA 004 Microbicide Trials', *AIDS* 26:123–6.

N.S. Padian (2010) 'Weighing the Gold in the Gold Standard: Challenges in HIV Prevention Research', Editorial Review *AIDS* 24:621–35.

N.S. Padian et al. (2007) 'Diaphragm and Lubricant Gel for Prevention of HIV Acquisition in Southern African Women: A Randomised Controlled Trial', *Lancet* 370:251–61.

N.S. Padian et al. (2008) 'Biomedical Interventions to Prevent HIV Infection: Evidence, Challenges, and Way Forward', *Lancet* 372:585–99.

N. S. Padian et al. (2011) 'HIV Prevention Transformed: The New Prevention Research Agenda', *Lancet* 378:269–78.

K. Page-Shafer et al. (2005) 'HIV Prevention Research in a Resource-limited Setting: The Experience of Planning a Trial in Cambodia', *Lancet* 366:1499–503.

C. Patton (1990) *Inventing AIDS* (New York and London: Routledge).

L. Paxton et al. (2007) 'Pre-exposure Prophylaxis for HIV Infection: What If It Works?', *Lancet* 370:89–93.

L. Paxton (2012) 'Considerations Regarding Antiretroviral Chemoprophylaxis and Heterosexuals in Generalized Epidemic Settings', *Current Opinion HIV AIDS* 7:557–62.

A.J.T.P. Peters et al. (2010) 'Where Does Public Funding for HIV Prevention Go To? The Case of Condoms versus Microbicides and Vaccines', *Globalization and Health* 6(23):1–10.

A. Petryna (2005) 'Ethical Variability: Drug Development and Globalizing Clinical Trials', *American Ethnologist* 32(2):183–97.

A. Petryna (2007) 'Clinical Trials Offshored: On Private Sector Science and Public Health', *BioSocieties* 2:21–40.

J. Phillips (2006) 'Agencement/Assemblage', *Theory, Culture and Society* 23:108–9.

J.V. Pickstone (2000) *Ways of Knowing: A New Science, Technology and Medicine* (Manchester: Manchester University Press).

L.C. Plein (1991) 'Popularising Biotechnology', *Science, Technology and Human Values* 16:474–90.

M. Poynten, I. Zablotska and A.E. Grulich (2012) 'Considerations Regarding Antiretroviral Chemoprophylaxis in MSM', *Current Opinion HIV AIDS* 7:549–56.

K. Race (2001) 'The Undetectable Crisis: Changing Technologies of Risk', *Sexualities* 4(2):167–89.

E. Richards and M. Ashmore (1996) 'More Sauce Please! The Politics of SSK: Neutrality, Commitment and Beyond', *Social Studies of Science* 26:219–28.

A. Rip (2002) 'Co-Evolution of Science, Technology and Society'. An Expert Review for the Bundesministerium Bildung und Forschung's Förderinitiative.

M. Rosengarten (2009) *HIV Interventions: Biomedicine and the Traffic in Information and Flesh* (Seattle, WA: University of Washington Press).

M. Rosengarten and M. Michael (2009a) 'Rethinking the Bioethical Enactment of Drugged Bodies: On the Paradoxes of Using Anti-HIV Drug Therapy as a Technology for Prevention', Special Issue on 'Living Drugs' *Science as Culture* 18(2):183–99.

M. Rosengarten and M. Michael (2009b) 'The Performative Function of Expectations in Translating Treatment to Prevention: The Case of HIV Pre-exposure Prophylaxis or PrEP', *Social Science & Medicine* 69(7):1049–55.

B. Salter and A. Faulker (2011) 'State strategies of governance in biomedical innovation: aligning conceptual approaches for understanding "Rising Powers" in the global context', *Globalization and Health* 7:3, available online at: http://demo.openrepository.com/demo/bitstream/2384/123193/1/Globalization%20and%20Health%202011.pdf [accessed 27 July 2011].

P.J.W. Saxton et al. (2012) 'Actual and undiagnosed HIV prevalence in a community sample of men who have sex with men in Auckland, New Zealand', *BMC Public Health* 12:92. Published online 2012 February 1. doi: 10.1186/1471-2458-12-92.

M. Serres (1982a) *Hermes: Literature, Science, Philosophy* (Baltimore, MA: Johns Hopkins University Press).

M. Serres (1982b) *The Parasite* (Baltimore, MA: Johns Hopkins University Press).

M. Serres and B. Latour (1995) *Conversations on Science, Culture and Time* (Ann Arbor, MI: Michigan University Press).

A. van Sighem et al. (2012) 'Resurgence of HIV Infection among Men Who Have Sex with Men in Switzerland: Mathematical Modelling Study', *PLoS ONE* 7(9):e44819.

S.D. Simon (2001) 'Is the Randomized Clinical Trial the Gold Standard of Research?', *Journal of Andrology* 22(6):938–43.

J.A. Singh and E.J. Mills (2005) 'The Abandoned Trials of Pre-Exposure Prophylaxis for HIV: What Went Wrong?', *PLoS Medicine* 2 (9, e234):0001–4.

M.K. Smith et al. (2012) HIV 'Treatment as Prevention: The Utility and Limitations of Ecological Observation', *PLoS Med* 9(7):e1001260, doi:10.1371/journal.pmed.1001260.

Z.A. Stein (1990) 'HIV Prevention: The Need for Methods Women Can Use', *American Journal of Public Health* 80:460–2.

I. Stengers (1997) 'Drugs: Ethical Choice or Moral Consensus' in *Power and Invention: Situating Science* (Minneapolis, MN and London: University of Minnesota Press).

I. Stengers (2000) *The Invention of Modern Science* (Minneapolis, MN: University of Minnesota Press).

I. Stengers (2005) 'The Cosmopolitical Proposal' in B. Latour and P. Webel (eds) *Making Things Public* (Cambridge, MA: MIT Press).

I. Stengers (2010) 'Including Nonhumans in Political Theory: Opening Pandora's Box' in B. Braun and S. J. Whatmore (eds) *Political Matter: Technoscience, Democracy and Public Life* (pp. 3–31) (Minneapolis, MN: University of Minnesota Press).

J. Stephenson and J. Imrie (1998) 'Why Do We Need Randomised Controlled Trials to Assess Behavioural Interventions?', *British Medical Journal* 316(7131):611–13.

J.M. Stephenson, J. Imrie and C. Bonell (eds) (2003) *Effective Sexual Health Interventions: Issues in Experimental Evaluation* (Oxford: Oxford University Press).

M. Strathern (1995) 'Cutting the Network', *Journal of the Royal Anthropological Institute (New Series)* 2: 517–35.

B. Szerszynski (2012) 'The Force of Experiment' Unpublished Manuscript.

TTATAG (The Thai AIDS Treatment Action Group) (2004) Letter 8 December, available at: http://www.aidsinfonyc.org/tag/activism/thaiTenofovir.html [accessed 9 June 2012].

M.C. Thigpen et al. (2012) 'Antiretroviral Preexposure Prophylaxis for Heterosexual HIV Transmission in Botswana', *New England Journal of Medicine* 367:423–34.

P.A. Thoits (1989) 'The Sociology of Emotions', *Annual Review of Sociology* 15: 317–42.

N. Thrift (2008) *Non-representational Theory* (London: Routledge).

F.J.W. Tomasini (2010) 'What is Bioethics: Notes towards a new approach?' *Studies in Ethics, Law and Technology* 4, 2, Article 7, available online at: http://www.bepress.com/selt/vol4/iss2/art7 [accessed 28 July 2011].

UNAIDS (2006) 'Creating effective partnerships for HIV prevention trials: report of a UNAIDS Consultation, Geneva 20–21 June 2005,' *AIDS* 20:W1–W11.

UNAIDS/WHO (2007) *Ethical considerations in biomedical HIV prevention trials* UNAIDS/WHO guidance document.

UNAIDS/AVAC (second edition 2011) *Good participatory practice: Guidelines for biomedical HIV prevention trials.*

UNAIDS (2012) 'Together we will end AIDS' (Joint United Nations Programme on HIV/AIDS).

UNFPA (2006) 'UNFPA: Working to Turn Back the AIDS Clock', available online at: http://www.unfpa.org/public/News/pid/228 -UNFPA [accessed 5 June 2012].

UNFPA (2012) 'About UNFPA', available online at: http://www.unfpa.org/public/home/about [accessed 29 November 2012].

L. Van Damme and M. Szpir (2012) 'Current Status of Topical Antiretroviral Chemoprophylaxis', *Current Opinion HIV AIDS* 7:520–5.

L. Van Damme et al. (2002) 'Effectiveness of COL-1492, a Nonoxynol-9 Vaginal Gel, on HIV-1 Transmission in Female Sex workers', *Lancet* 360:970–7.

L. Van Damme et al. (2012) 'Preexposure Prophylaxis for HIV Infection among African Women', *New England Journal of Medicine* 367:411–22.

A. Van der Zaag [unpublished doctoral thesis] 'The Promise of Vaginal Microbicides: Configurations of Women's Empowerment in a Time of HIV' Department of Sociology, Goldsmiths, University of London.

A. Webster (2002) 'Innovative Health Technologies and the Social: Redefining Health, Medicine and the Body', *Current Sociology* 50:443–57.

A.N. Whitehead (1978) *Process and Reality. An Essay in Cosmology* (New York: The Free Press).

WHO/UNAIDS (2004) 'Treating people with intercurrent infection in HIV prevention trials: report from A WHO/UNAIDS consultation, Geneva 17–18 July 2003', *AIDS* 18:W1–W12.

WHO (World Health Organization) (2012a) 'Voluntary medical male circumcision for HIV prevention' Fact sheet: July. http://www.who.int/hiv/topics/malecircumcision/fact_sheet/en/index.html [accessed 6 October 2012].

WHO (2012b) Guidance on Pre-exposure Oral Prophylaxis (PrEP) for Serodiscordant Couples, Men and Transgender Women Who Have Sex with Men at High Risk of HIV: Recommendations for Use in the Context of Demonstration Projects (published by WHO).

C. Will and T. Moreira (2010) 'Introduction' in C. Will and T. Moreira (eds) *Medical Proofs, Social Experiments: Clinical Trials in Shifting Contexts* (Farnham: Ashgate).

WNU (Women's Network for Unity) (2004) Protests Drug Trial Recruitment Tactics, 15 June. Public statement released by WNU Secretariat.

C. Woodsong and Q.A. Karim (2005) 'Experiences from the HIV Prevention Trials Network', *American Journal of Public Health* 95(3):412–19.

C. Woodsong et al. (2006) 'Women's Autonomy and Informed Consent in International Microbicide Clinical Trials', *Journal of Empirical Research on Human Research Ethics* 1556–2646:11–26.

B.E. Wynne (1989). 'Frameworks of Rationality in Risk Management: Towards the Testing of Naive Sociology' in J. Brown (ed.) *Environmental Threats* (pp. 33–47) (London: Belhaven Press).

B.E. Wynne (1995) 'The Public Understanding of Science' in S. Jasanoff et al. (eds) *Handbook of Science and Technology Studies* (pp. 361–88) (Thousand Oaks, CA: Sage).

B.E. Wynne (2006) 'Public Engagement as a Means of Restoring Public Trust in Science – Hitting the Notes, but Missing the Music?', *Public Health Genomics* 9:211–20.

Index